Expressive Arts Therapy
Creative Process in Art and Life

Appalachian Expressive Arts Collective

Sally Atkins
Marianne Adams
Cathy McKinney
Harold McKinney
Liz Rose
Jay Wentworth
Joan Woodworth

Sharon Sharp, Editor
Kathy Isaacs, Editorial Assistant, Hubbard Center

Parkway Publishers, Inc.
Boone, North Carolina

Parkway
Publishers
© 2003

Expressive arts therapy : creative process in art and life/Appalachian
Expressive Arts Collective ; Sally Atkins ... [et al.].

    p. cm.

Includes bibliographical references.

  ISBN 1-887905-68-5

  1. Arts—Therapeutic use. I. Atkins, Sally S. II. Appalachian
Expressive Arts Collective.

  RC489.A72 E97 2002

  615.8'515—dc21

  2002009498

Typesetting: Kathy Isaacs; Beth Jacquot

Cover Design: Shuntavia Graham

Front Cover Art: Sally Atkins, "Deepest Impulse"

Back Cover Photo: Mike Rominger

Dedication

This is a book of many voices,
an
ensemble.

It includes the voices of
our colleagues, our families, our clients,
and, especially
our students.

It is to them this book is dedicated
in deep appreciation of their inspiration and energy
for our collective learning.

—The Appalachian Expressive Arts Collective

Acknowledgements

Many people deserve our sincere thanks for their help and support in the creation of this book. Our colleagues in the academic departments of Human Development and Psychological Counseling, Interdisciplinary Studies, Psychology, Theatre and Dance, and the School of Music at Appalachian State University have supported and nurtured our creative expression in many ways.

We are grateful to the Hubbard Center for Faculty and Staff Support for their initial funding of this project. Thanks go to Kate Brinko who inspired us to undertake interdisciplinary work in a formal way and continually encouraged and supported us through many difficulties. We are grateful to Kathy Isaacs for her creative wisdom in the formatting and design of the book. We would like to thank our graduate assistants, Mary Beth Rabon and Jill Masten-Byers, for their valuable assistance with this project. Special thanks go to Scarlet Tison, who spent hours keyboarding editorial changes with grace and goodwill, and to Laurie Atkins, who did innumerable tasks and errands and helped with the artwork.

We are grateful to the Blumenthal Foundation for the opportunity to be Writers in Residence at Wildacres Retreat, where a great deal of the work of this project was done. Thanks go to Philip Blumenthal, Mike House, and the staff of Wildacres for creating a space where we could live and work in a true expressive arts community.

We wish to thank several colleagues in the international community of expressive arts, who offered comments, suggestions, challenges, and support, which have helped us to shape our unique perspective on this emerging field. Thanks go to Juergen Kriz, Herbert Eberhart, Majken Jacoby, Margo Fuchs, Shawn McNiff, Steen Lykke, and Stephen and Ellen Levine, all faculty members at the European Graduate School in Switzerland. Particular thanks go to Paolo Knill, Provost of the European Graduate School, for his leadership in the field and for his ongoing inspiration and friendship.

We would like to acknowledge those teachers and artists, too many to name, who have inspired us and furthered our growth. In the field of expressive arts therapy and in our respective disciplines of counseling, psychology, music, dance, and creative writing, we have been gifted with many mentors. The opinions expressed in this book, of course, remain those of the authors.

Finally, we are grateful to each other. We are grateful for the opportunity to participate in a truly collaborative project of creative expression, to live the ideas and practices about which we are speaking.

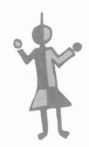

CONTENTS

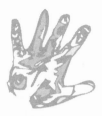

INTRODUCTION

The Expressive Arts Collective at Appalachian State University had its inception in 1985 when the Department of Human Development and Psychological Counseling first offered a course, Therapy and the Expressive Arts. Faculty presenters included counselors, arts therapists, therapists who were artists, and artists who used dreams and the creative process for personal and professional growth. In August 1997, five faculty members who had been collaborating in that course began to meet monthly, thereby establishing a formal interdisciplinary collective of faculty interested in expressive arts. The purpose of the collective was to share expertise, seek additional training, work together in informal team teaching, and develop an integrative expressive arts emphasis within the master's degree program in counseling. The book, Expressive Arts: An Invitation to the Journey, was one product of that first year's work.

Since that time, the collective has continued to meet monthly, teach collaboratively, participate in training, and offer an annual experiential institute in expressive arts therapy. New members have joined, expanding the group to represent five departments in four colleges of the university. The work of the expanded Collective resulted in a second book, entitled *Collective Voices* in Expressive Arts. This third book, *Expressive Arts Therapy: Creative Process in Art and Life*, is an outgrowth of our continuing collaborative work, with each other and with our students.

The preparation of this book has required immersion by the authors in the same process about which we write—moving into that deep sacred space from which creativity springs and emerging to share our findings in community. We have encountered the same types of experiences as in any therapeutic or creative process, including the need to clear space, find focus, and center ourselves; the resistance to and fear of moving into the work; the taste of shadow and the touch of light in the depths of the work; the struggle to name that which we have experienced; and the challenge to apply that which we are learning in our individual and collective outer lives.

Working together to prepare this book has brought tremendous blessings. Although our progress sometimes has seemed glacially slow, the product of this pentimento process has been richer. We have been inspired and energized by working together. Our collective wisdom is exponentially stronger than that of any one of us. For some, this work has connected and legitimized threads in our lives that have lain in disparate corners. For others, it has enriched artistic endeavors by keeping us aware of the importance of connection with the art, with the audience, and with ourselves. For all of us, it is a sacred privilege to work in an intimate community of scholar-teacher-therapists who not only share common interests, but who also have experienced deepening through personal adversity and have the courage to share that process with others.

This book is written primarily for therapists and for students who are becoming therapists. We hope that it may also prove insightful to artists, teachers, and others interested in exploring the power of expressive arts for growth and healing. It offers theoretical grounding and practical applications that have grown from our collective experience. The book is a synthesis of our training and experience in our disciplines and our collective journey in expressive arts.

Part 1

FOUNDATIONS

Expressive arts therapy is a new and emerging field within psychotherapeutic practice. In part 1 we describe our perspectives on the historical context and theoretical grounding for this emerging field.

In chapter 1 we introduce expressive arts therapy as a reclaiming of ancient traditions that combined community, ritual, and art in healing. We also situate expressive arts therapy within the context of psychological theory and provide a brief overview of the historical development and current practice in the field. The chapter concludes with our collective view of the major premises of our approach to expressive arts therapy and our view of expressive arts therapy as an interdisciplinary and integrative paradigm.

In chapter 2 we focus on the practice of expressive arts therapy. We highlight the therapist's ability to serve as a facilitator of creative process and a witness to the work of art making. Finally, we emphasize the importance of the personal integrity and ongoing growth of the therapist, and we offer some special considerations for the artist-therapist working in this field.

Many voices contribute to the richness and variety of views and practice within the field of expressive arts. Our views are shaped by our differing disciplinary backgrounds in counseling, psychology, dance, music, music therapy, poetry, philosophy, theology, and interdisciplinary studies. We also are influenced by many years of professional practice as teachers, therapists, and artists.

We must add that our views about expressive arts, therapy, and life are also inextricably linked with the natural landscape in which we live. We live and work in the ancient mountains of the Southern Appalachian Range, among remnants of the oldest forests on earth, at the birthplace of four rivers, including the oldest river on the continent of North America. This is the landscape that shapes our daily life and inhabits our souls.

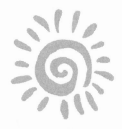

Chapter 1

EXPRESSIVE ARTS THERAPY: AN EVOLVING FIELD

We live in a time and in a culture in which the arts have become separated from the day-to-day lives of ordinary people. Artists, musicians, dancers, and writers are those who have received highly specialized training or those who have become commercially successful with their artistic productions. Works of art often live in galleries, museums, and theaters, but not in the daily lives of human beings. Healing practices, too, have been separated from the purview of ordinary life and are usually performed by highly specialized practitioners, trained in the latest methods of modern science.

The integrated use of the arts is ancient. It harks back to times when ceremonies of birth and death, marriage and coming of age, planting and harvesting, as well as rituals of spiritual, mental, and physical healing, all involved the arts. Ancient peoples sang and danced, beat drums, made images, and told stories to celebrate and mourn the passages of life, to find their place in relationship with each other, and to remember and honor their relationship with the natural world. The healing practices of indigenous cultures around the world unite creative expression and healing. In such cultures, healing practices reflect an integrated scientific, philosophical, and spiritual consciousness.

Expressive arts therapy—also referred to as intermodal expressive therapy, creative arts therapy, or interdisciplinary arts therapy—is the practice of using imagery, storytelling, dance, music, drama, poetry, movement, dreamwork, and visual arts together, in an integrated way, to foster human growth, development, and healing. It is about reclaiming our innate capacity as human beings for creative expression of our individual and collective human experience in artistic form. Expressive arts therapy is also about experiencing the natural capacity of creative expression and creative community for healing. (See Plate #1.)

Historical Development

Interdisciplinary expressive arts therapy is a relatively new and rapidly expanding field in therapeutic practice. While evolving, the different specific arts therapies have usually been separated from one another and have been organized around specific mediums or modalities. Each arts therapy has developed its own formal clinical training, usually at the graduate level, and a tradition of individual apprenticeship training and credentialing. Fields such as art therapy, music therapy, dance/movement therapy, poetry therapy, and psychodrama have existed for some time, and some have their own journals and professional organizations, such as the American Art Therapy Association, the American Dance Therapy Association, the American Music Therapy Association, the American Association of Group Psychotherapy and Psychodrama, the National Association for Drama Therapy, the National Association for Poetry Therapy, and the Association for the Study of Dreams. Most have ethical guidelines, standards of practice, and registration or certification procedures. Some of the specific arts therapies have operated within the traditional medical model of illness and cure and within psychodynamic models of psychotherapy. By contrast, expressive arts therapy is interdisciplinary and holistic, grounded more in theories of existential phenomenology, depth psychology, humanistic psychotherapy, and systems theories.

In the early 1970s, Shaun McNiff, Paolo Knill, Norma Canner, and their colleagues founded the Expressive Therapies Program at Lesley College Graduate School, now Leslie University, in Cambridge, Massachusetts. This program emphasized an interdisciplinary, intermodal approach to arts therapy and the formation of a creative, therapeutic community of students and faculty. In the 1980s Paolo Knill developed a network of training programs in Europe and North America under the title of the International School of Interdisciplinary Studies. A number of these training institutes now exist around the world. Many academic institutions also offer training in expressive arts as a part of programs in counseling and therapy, and doctoral programs in expressive arts therapy are offered by the European Graduate School in Switzerland and Leslie University.

In addition to the formation of training programs, a number of other factors have influenced the emergence of this field. Since 1985 the National Coalition of Arts Therapies Associations has encouraged cross-disciplinary communication and sharing among the individual arts therapies. The establishment of the journal *The Arts in Psychotherapy* has fostered interdisciplinary learning among the arts, as will the newly established journal *Poesis: A Journal of the Arts and Communication*. Within the American Psychological Association, the Psychology and the Arts Division (Division 10) continues to increase awareness of creative arts approaches in the field of psychology. The International Expressive Arts Therapy Association, formed in 1994, is a major contributor to the development of the profession. This organization has sponsored several major conferences in the United States and Canada and has begun a professional registration process for expressive arts therapists.

Current Contributors to the Field of Expressive Arts Therapy

Many artists, clinicians, theoreticians, and philosophers continue to define the practice of expressive arts therapy. Some colleagues who have contributed to our current understanding of the field are Shaun McNiff, Paolo Knill, Margo Fuchs, Majken Jacoby, Herbert Eberhart, Juergen Kriz, Margo Fuchs, Elizabeth McKim, Yaacov Naor, Geoffrey Scott-Alexander, Stephen and Ellen Levine, all faculty members of the European Graduate School in Switzerland.

Shaun McNiff, of Leslie University, has made major contributions to the literature on the education, theory, and practice of expressive arts therapy. Key ideas from his writing include the importance of honoring the images of art (by listening to them rather than analyzing or interpreting them) and the interdependence of diverse disciplines and their natural integration into expressive arts therapy. McNiff asserts that the expansion of the creative arts therapy profession can be attributed largely to a primal (and not always conscious) longing for the integration of the essential elements of the healing process. He suggests that creativity should become a major health concept (McNiff, 1986, 1989, 1992, 1998). He also acknowledges the universal and cross-cultural elements of creativity and healing and suggests strong societal implications for their integration. "The creative arts therapies in their most enlightened and liberating forms are indicating a new vision of art in society, which suggests the restoration of an ancient and archetypal integration of the creative process with healing" (McNiff, 1986, p. 5).

Paolo Knill, the provost of the European Graduate School and an internationally beloved teacher in expressive arts, articulates principles of intermodal work using two theoretical frameworks to explain the paradoxical nature of expressive arts therapy. The theory of polyaesthetics emphasizes the understanding of the arts as distinct, yet interconnected. Crystallization theory, as applied to expressive arts, relates to the human yearning to articulate the essence of human experience, to find meaning by giving form to experience through different arts disciplines. Knill emphasizes aesthetic response and response-ability as important elements in intermodal work (Knill et al., 1995).

Stephen and Ellen Levine, founders of ISIS-Canada and co-editors of *Foundations of Expressive Arts Therapy* (1999) combine poetry, drama, and visual art in expressive arts therapy. Stephen is a founder of the International Expressive Arts Therapy Association and editor of *Poiesis: A Journal of the Arts and Communication*. He situates expressive arts therapy within the philosophical traditions of Kant and Heidegger and sees the imagination, the realm of creativity, as an essential feature of our human existence, our way of shaping and claiming authentic relationship to the world (Levine, 1992, 1999, 2000). Ellen Levine, a visual artist and therapist, writes, teaches, supervises, and practices in the areas of play and expressive arts therapy. Her writings reflect her personal and professional experience in expressive arts therapy, grounded in psychoanalytic theory. She combines personal, theoretical, and clinical material, centering on the idea of creative expression as an internal fire, a life force in the self (Levine, 1995).

Other faculty members of the European Graduate School who have made important contributions to our thinking include Majken Jacoby, Herbert Eberhart, Juergen Kriz, Geoffrey Scott-Alexander, Margo Fuchs, and Elizabeth McKim. Majken Jacoby emphasizes the importance of both ethics and aesthetics in expressive arts therapy. She points to the ethical demand for us as human beings to take care of and give form to the life we hold in our hands, the life that is given to us. The "necessity of form" as an act of care is, for Jacoby (2000), the core of expressive arts. Herbert Eberhart (2001) emphasizes the importance of therapeutic presence in expressive arts. The work of the therapist is to be fully present in an open way to the other person and to the artistic experience. Eberhart's presence is a careful and sensitive attentiveness, one that he lives as well as teaches. Juergen Kriz (2001) is a primary contributor to the field of expressive arts therapy in the areas of phenomenological psychology, self-organization and systems theory, and research. Yaacov Naor (1999) works in the area of psychodrama to demonstrate the therapeutic theater is an arena in which conflict and pain can be contained and confronted. He works with Israelis and Palestinians, with children of Jewish survivors of the Holocaust and children of German parents of World War II. Geoffrey Scott-Alexander is a body-centered expressive arts therapist. Using his background in theatre, body work, and expressive arts therapy, he emphasizes centeredness and openheartedness in a contemplative expressive arts practice. Margo Fuchs and Elizabeth McKim are poets of the expressive arts. Fuchs sees poetry as a way of knowing, poetry and image as ways the soul reveals itself beyond the boundaries of rational logic (Fuchs, 1996). McKim reminds us that poetry originates in primal rhythm and rhyme, that poetic language is part of our inheritance, the ability to shape experience with words (McKim, 1999).

Other pioneers in expressive arts whose work we have studied are Natalie Rogers, Anna Halprin, and Daria Halprin Khaligeri. Natalie Rogers, founder of the Person-Centered Expressive Therapy Training Institute in California, has developed her approach with reference to the person-centered theory developed by her father, Carl Rogers. Her method is called the "creative connection," emphasizing the process of allowing one art form to influence another directly. She emphasizes process over product and trusting in the client's capacity to make personal meaning of images and symbols. (Rogers, 1993). The work of Anna Halprin and her daughter, Daria Halprin Kalighi, in dance, movement, theater, and ritual is an inspiring example of the use of the arts and the natural world for healing. Their work at Talmalpa Institute in California and around the world has continued to explore movement and ritual for a variety of healing purposes, from reconnecting with the earth to dealing with AIDS (Halprin, 1995; Halprin Kalighi, 1989).

Other contributions toward this emerging field have included writings from the literature of counseling and psychotherapy, the literature of creativity and the creative process, and the literature of specific arts therapies. Many of these that we have found most useful are included by category in the Bibliography. A few of these writings have been so influential in our thinking that we wish to highlight them.

Many mental health professionals use various arts activities in assessment or therapy, but not necessarily as a primary method or in a systematic way. In *Beyond Talk Therapy*, Daniel Wiener (1999), a psychologist, marriage and family therapist, and professor at Central Connecticut University, introduces a selection of "action methods" and creative approaches to psychotherapy. Weiner defines action methods as those that engage the client in purposeful physical activity, such as expressive arts, movement, and enactment. Wiener acknowledges that psychotherapy will continue to be a verbally mediated process, but he asserts that such action methods can be integral to and effective in therapy.

Sam Gladding, a national leader in the fields of counseling and poetry therapy, and a professor at Wake Forest University, has provided a great deal of information on how various creative arts can be used both independently and complementarily in the counseling process. Through his many books and articles, Gladding has argued effectively for an expansion of the use of creative arts in the field of counseling. He asserts that all good counseling employs an artistic quality that enables clients to express themselves in a creative and unique way. He points out that "by engaging in the playful, cooperative, and communicative dimensions of art, individuals recognize more clearly the complexity and simplicity of their lives" (1998, p. 11).

Within the literature on creativity, we must make special note of the work of M. C. Richards and Steven Nachmanovitch. Richards, a potter and poet, was a member of the experimental community of artists at Black Mountain College. Her work provides a richly poetic and deeply philosophical grounding for an understanding of the intimate relationship between the arts and healing. In *Centering: In Poetry, Pottery, and the Person*, Richards (1989) calls for the integration of art, mysticism, and community within a living cosmology. Her themes include the union of opposites in the quest for understanding self and universe, and the need for moral courage and compassion. She reminds us that the artist's way of knowing is that of perception, so we must be about the awakening, cleansing, and reverencing of perception. Perception is not a concept but an experience of nature. It is essential, says Richards, to enter into these artistic explorations from the inside, or they become only decorative tricks. The focus is not on the effect, but on the feeling that precedes the act (Richards, 1966, 1989, 1996).

In *Free Play: The Power of Improvisation in Life and the Arts*, the musician, poet, and teacher, Steven Nachmanovitch (1990) explores the playful nature of creativity. He views all of the arts and life as improvisational and sees the heart of improvisation as the free play of consciousness. According to Nachmanovitch, the basis for accessing creativity and improvisation is play: "Play is the taproot from which original art springs" (p. 42). He suggests the creative process as a spiritual path and explores the joy and peace, as well as the understanding and responsibility, that come from the full use of human imagination.

Many contributions to expressive arts therapy have been made from practitioners and theorists in the specialized arts fields. Contributions from the fields of music therapy, arts therapy, and dreamwork include those of Helen Bonny, Carolyn Kenny, Pat Allen, Margaret Keyes, Peter London, and Jill Mellick.

While many music therapists have employed multi-arts experiences within their clinical practices, Helen Bonny and Carolyn Kenny have made significant methodological and theoretical contributions to the use of expressive arts in therapy. As a pioneer in the use of music, imagery, altered states of consciousness, and mandalas in the Bonny Method of Guided Imagery and Music, Helen Bonny (1978a, 1978b; Bonny & Savary, 1990) has contributed significantly to our understanding of the potential for self-exploration, healing, and transformation through receptive immersion in music and imagery. Carolyn Kenny (1982) was among the first to describe integrated arts experiences in therapy, and she has also offered a theoretical model unique to therapeutic experiences in music (Kenny, 1989).

Significant contributions to expressive arts therapy from the visual arts include those of Pat Allen, Margaret Keyes, and Peter London. In *Art as a Way of Knowing*, Pat Allen (1995) suggests that art making is both a spiritual practice and a way of knowing. She says that giving form to the images of our dreams, imagination, and daily lives is a type of spiritual practice that leads to self-knowledge and wisdom. She offers personal stories and insights, as well as practical suggestions for methods and activities. Margaret Keyes (1983) presents varied techniques of painting, sculpture, music, and story in *Inward Journey*. Focusing on Jungian and Gestalt principles, she makes explicit her view of using art materials for self-understanding, rather than for diagnosis and treatment of disease. Her techniques involve the art experience itself, as well as an emphasis on a meditation process. "An art experience in itself can be powerfully healing when one is fully engrossed with the materials and the process" (p. vii). In *No More Second Hand Art*, Peter London (1989) has emphasized that art is about much more than decoration, innovation, and self-expression. He speaks of the transformative capacity of the creative process in personal growth and empowerment and in communion with the world. London calls for the reclaiming of visual image making as a natural form of expression for every person.

Many practitioners, therapists, and researchers in the field of dreamwork make use of expressive forms, especially enactment and visual arts in working with dreams. Jill Mellick (1996), in *The Natural Artistry of Dreams*, sees dreams as an expression of the natural creative process of the dreamer and emphasizes the use of expressive arts modalities as primary vehicles for exploring the meaning of dreams.

There are many other current pioneers whose practice and writings will continue to shape this rapidly expanding field. Mental health practitioners, artists, and arts therapists who work in integrative and collaborative ways will contribute to a broader understanding of interdisciplinary art making as healing. As a work in progress, expressive arts therapy will continue to define itself as an emerging paradigm.

Expressive Arts Therapy and Psychotherapy

Our approach to expressive arts is grounded in the practice of art-making and creative expression as a means of giving form to the essential experiences of life. Our use of expressive arts as a therapeutic practice is based on interdisciplinary collaborative process and draws from a foundation in psychotherapeutic theory.

From psychoanalytic and neopsychoanalytic theories of psychotherapy, expressive arts therapy draws on the concept of the unconscious mind as a storehouse of rich knowledge (Freud, 1940). Our practice of expressive arts therapy also draws from

Jungian psychology, with its emphasis on the existence of universal cross-cultural archetypes, myths, and symbols in the collective unconscious. Also important are creativity and spirituality in personal growth and healing, and the use of dreamwork and creative expression as a means of accessing the deep wisdom and healing capacities of the unconscious mind (Jung, 1964).

The primary contribution of behavioral psychotherapy to expressive arts is a substantial body of research supporting the efficacy of consciousness-altering methods of relaxation and guided imagery for the relief of stress and anxiety (Wolpe, 1958). In our practice of expressive arts therapy, we use ritual, poetry, music, and artmaking, as well as other methods of breathwork, movement, and imagining to create a focused state in which therapeutic work can be done.

From the humanistic and existential psychotherapies, especially from the person-centered therapy of Carol Rogers (1961), our philosophy of expressive arts therapy draws the concept of an innate, creative, positive striving capacity in human nature. From this perspective, personal growth and creativity are the natural tendencies of human beings, especially given an environment that supports and nurtures such growth (Maslow, 1962; May, 1975; Perls, 1973; Rogers, 1961; Zinker, 1978).

Contributions from systems theorists to the field of expressive arts therapy include an awareness of the importance of context and an understanding of the individual as a part of complex, interacting, and self organizing systems, whether family groups, larger communities, or the natural world (von Bertanlanffy, 1968; Bowen, 1978; Minuchin, 1974; Satir, 1972; Sullivan, 1953; Whitaker & Bumberry, 1988). We see the therapist as acting and being acted upon in the therapeutic process within a social and cultural context.

Within the disciplines of psychology and counseling, expressive arts therapy is a new, emerging, and integrative practice. For the most part, the discipline of psychology is situated squarely within the objectivist, materialist worldview of Western science. Behavioral, physiological, and cognitive approaches to psychology share the assumptions of classical Western science, which emphasize objectivism, reductionism, materialism, and determinism in understanding human behavior. The therapeutic practices that have emerged from this worldview emphasize the diagnosis and treatment of human problems as dysfunction and disease. Over the last several decades, the adequacy of these assumptions for understanding human experience and healing have been challenged with increasing vigor. Scientists and nonscientists alike have argued for the necessity of a shift to a more holistic and purposive approach to science that values subjectivity, inner experience, and the unity of body, mind, and spirit (Capra, 1996; Harman, 1994; Peat, 1991; Tarnas, 1991). Further, cultural changes in society have suggested the need to rediscover the spiritual aspects of human experience (Harman, 1994).

Expressive arts therapy suggests new concepts and raises new questions about the nature of being human, the meaning of human suffering, and the nature of personal change and of psychological and spiritual growth. Expressive arts therapy celebrates connectedness, deep feeling, creativity, intuition, integration, purpose, and the totality of the human experience.

Premises within Expressive Arts Therapy
The Appalachian School

In reviewing key literature and in examining our own collective principles from our respective professional backgrounds and experience, we suggest that our current practice in expressive arts therapy is rooted in the following premises:

- Expressive arts therapy, as we practice it, is a collaborative process. It is a collaboration between therapist and client, scientist and artist, teacher and student. It acknowledges that all participants bring an equal voice to the conversation and make a valued contribution to the work.

- Expressive arts therapy is holistic. Its goals are optimum health and well-being, rather than the diagnosis and treatment of disease and dysfunction. Even when expressive arts are used within the settings of traditional medical and psychological treatment, they are used in service of learning, healing, and growth.

- Art making and creative expression are healing, growth-producing processes in and of themselves, not adjunctive to traditional therapy. While reflection on process and product may be part of the work, the emphasis remains on the capacity for therapeutic transformation inherent in giving form to creative expression.

- The capacity for creative expression is a fundamental aspect of health. Thus, healing and personal growth are possible through involvement in the creative process.

- In expressive arts therapy, body knowledge, intuitive wisdom, subjective experience, and emotions are expressed and honored as valid ways of knowing in and of themselves. Rational analysis is not required to validate them.

- Expressive arts therapy is depth-oriented. Work in the arts provides access to emotions, experiences, and insights not often reached through traditional psychological practice. Such work provides powerful access to unconscious material.

- Expressive arts therapy often involves the layering of modalities. Like all interdisciplinary work, it enlarges the capacity of both the client and the therapist to hold different perspectives, to speak many "languages" simultaneously.

- The integrity of an expressive arts therapist is reflected in ongoing personal use of creative expression for personal healing and growth. While the therapist may have expertise in one artistic modality, she seeks personal experiences in other modalities.

- Expressive arts therapy, because of its emphasis on community and ritual, suggests the reclaiming of an ancient vision of art and therapy in society, one that integrates art and healing in the context of community. This vision suggests that art and therapy and life are not separate, and that all are practiced in community for the healing of both the individual and the community as a whole.

- In its broadest and deepest sense, expressive arts therapy is a spiritual practice. It offers the possibility for meditative practice and for entry into what may be described as an experience of universal consciousness.

The role of creativity in healing, the reclaiming of the natural artistic capacity of human beings, and the integrated use of the expressive arts in therapy increasingly have become topics of interest and importance to individuals and to our society. The field of expressive arts therapy is a dynamic and rapidly expanding area of mental health practice. The literature of the field will continue to expand as more artists and practitioners contribute to the collective conversation about these ideas.

Chapter 2

THE PRACTICE OF
EXPRESSIVE ARTS THERAPY

*T*he practice of expressive arts therapy is shaped by the therapist's ideas about what it means to be a human being, the nature of creativity, human growth and development, and human suffering. If we accept the premise that growth, creative expression, and healing are natural processes, then the role of the therapist centers upon affirming and supporting those natural processes rather than analyzing, diagnosing, or fixing.

The Therapeutic Relationship

The foundation of all psychotherapeutic practice is the ground of relationship. We begin with experiencing our basic human connection—being fully present in the moment together, listening deeply to what is said, what is left unspoken, and what is spoken without awareness. We pay close attention to the language of the body, the client's and our own. By allowing the experience of connection to deepen, accepting and honoring who we are, at that moment, with all our limits, flaws, and imperfections, we provide an opportunity for the client to feel seen, heard, and understood without judgment. As we experience our shared vulnerability, intimacy and trust develop between us, and we make a space together that is safe and sacred, a place where truth-telling, growth, and healing can occur, a place where deep wisdom can be recognized. The authentic presence of the therapist is the most significant factor in the creation of a therapeutic relationship.

Bearing Witness to Story

The work of the therapist is to bear witness to the beauty, ugliness, pain, suffering, and joy of the human story. The recognition of the self by another, the experience of connection with each other's stories at a soul level is profoundly healing and transformative for both client and therapist. For the expressive arts therapist, the human story is revealed in narrative form but also in poetic images and in languages that are not words—in movement, music, and visual forms. Thus the therapist is called upon to respond to the artistic products, as well as the creative process, of the client.

Facilitative responses to artistic expression may include purely literal descriptions of what is seen and heard. Sometimes what is needed is the ability to mirror or reflect just what is there, to simply articulate what we see or hear, not to fix, suggest, or critique. This type of reflection allows the creator to understand the clarity and intention expressed in her own work and to take in the information offered at many different levels.

The therapist's response should facilitate the movement of both client and therapist more deeply into the therapeutic and creative processes. Aesthetic responses—acknowledging how the responder is touched personally by the work—in words or in creative forms can be helpful. We must remember that such images, body responses, emotions, and memories belong to the responder, and they provide a means of acknowledging our deep human connections with each other.

One of the most powerful ways of responding to aesthetic works is silence. Silence deep enough to hold the full presence of the therapist, the client, and the work can be a holy space, beyond words, which allows for the entrance of the sacred—however we name the forces larger than our little selves.

The experience of "standing to"—that is, owning, acknowledging, and revealing—the truth of one's own experience is itself a powerful vehicle for healing and growth. To have that personal truth witnessed by another and to experience an inner resonance of mutual understanding is to affirm that we, as human beings, are deeply touched by truth, honesty, and integrity. As expressive arts therapists, we are privileged to witness that expressions of truth are exquisitely beautiful, even when they are not pretty.

Therapeutic Process

All therapy involves facilitating the creative process. The therapist nurtures the basic life force energy, affirms the client's capacity to change, and encourages new attitudes and possibilities. The expressive arts therapist honors the power of the creative process and uses this process directly in a variety of ways to encourage growth. We make a space of freedom and playfulness, full of choice and inspiration, like a preschool teacher who honors play as a wellspring for creativity and who offers clay, paints, crayons, and music and simply allows expression, without product in mind, but for the profound purpose of creating.

The process of therapy involves deepening the questions we are asking about our lives. Because each person harbors a memory of his or her wiser, more knowing (and imperfect) self, the work of therapy is also about remembering and affirming who we are at the deepest level. It is also about re-membering ourselves—working to integrate seemingly disparate parts of the self. We honor the experience of dis-integration and integration as part of a natural cycle. Dis-integration—a sense of coming apart, intrapersonally or interpersonally—is often what brings a person to therapy. The expressive arts therapist sees this not as a symptom to be alleviated but as a part of the natural cycle and, thus, an opportunity for growth.

The expressive arts therapist understands and uses the arts to bring to bear all the senses, the body as a whole, emotion, intuition, dreams, visions, expressive skills, and intelligence to support the client's natural movement toward meaning making and wholeness. In the process, the client may feel increased tension, emotional shifts, or a sense of letting go of old habits; all of these are signs of personal growth. In moments of integration there is often a release of tension, a flood of emotion, or an intellectual "ah-ha!"

The work of expressive arts therapy often leads us to our own growing edge, that place where knowledge is new and not completely comfortable. It is a place of risk and freedom. Without fresh insight that springs from the unconscious soul, stagnation occurs. The artistry and challenge of the therapist are to be with the client as he moves through the cycle of preparing, creating, reflecting, and then living each piece of art. Ultimately, our role as therapists is about our ability to be present on an unpredictable journey, with no road maps and no final destinations.

One of the greatest challenges for the therapist is timing—knowing when and how to challenge, support, build safety nets, hold and cradle, cajole, wait patiently, interject humor, or merely have the sense to get out of the way. Knowing when to take which approach comes from careful listening and experience, and even then is an imperfect art. The ability to ask questions that facilitate the client's movement toward deeper awareness and understanding is the mark of a great therapist. Asking questions of vision and depth is a skill that cannot be taught and must be finely honed from clinical experience.

The Person of the Therapist

Competent practice in expressive arts therapy requires the therapist to have knowledge of individual personality organization, understanding of individual and group process dynamics, skills in facilitating therapeutic growth, and personal experience with a variety of arts modalities. Knowing how to structure arts media into therapeutic experiences comes from our own self-exploration and growth. It is a way of knowing from the inside out.

Beyond knowledge and skills, the therapist's genuineness and integrity are essential elements in every psychotherapeutic process. The desire for integrity motivates the therapist's daily art and spiritual practice. We consciously pursue "daily practice" in order to center ourselves and prepare to enter creative space with clients. We are constantly involved in our own process of development as artists, as therapists, and as human beings.

Special Considerations

To be human is to be creative. All people have the capacity to enjoy and experience growth through creative expression. However, expressive methods are powerful and must be used with great sensitivity to the developmental stage, personality organization, and interpersonal dynamics of clients. Some groups or individuals require special consideration by a facilitator of expressive arts experiences.

In many expressive arts practices, the combination of ritual and inward focus leads to a state of consciousness that is different from our everyday active, alert state. For many of us, it is this non-ordinary state of consciousness that allows us to tap deeply into our own psyches to access insights, wisdom, and life-altering experiences. These inward-focused, meditative states can be powerful tools for growth and healing.

For young children, the creation of a non-ordinary state of consciousness is unnecessary. Children naturally function in a more holistic, less linear way than do most adults. Absorption in play and creative expression is as natural for them as breath. The therapist or facilitator need provide little more than appropriate media and opportunity for natural creative expression to occur.

For some persons, encouragement of a more internally focused state of consciousness is contraindicated. The altered state increases the permeability of the boundary that most of us recognize between imaginal events and events in our external lives. Individuals with psychosis or other psychologically fragile conditions already may have little or no boundary between internal and external events. They may have difficulty returning from an intense internal experience to ordinary functioning in external reality. For both of these groups, adaptations to the way of working may be required. Shorter time frames may be appropriate, and the experience may be designed to encourage a more external focus. For example, participants may be encouraged to talk aloud during visual arts experiences such as working with clay or collage. Experiences with music may invite participants to move or draw to music, rather than silently form images. The music itself may be shorter, more inherently structured, and less emotionally evocative than that which is appropriate for adults with well-established defenses.

Immersion in expressive arts experiences may more easily bypass defenses than does traditional verbal therapy. Because of this, the facilitator of such experiences must take care to move into experiences slowly, making sure to prepare the way and establish safety, especially in groups.

Closure is important in all forms of therapy, but especially so in therapies that work in alternative states of consciousness. At the end of each session, it is the therapist's responsibility to ascertain whether the participant is ready to reenter the world, since the person in the altered state may be able to accurately judge that only in retrospect. Moving the conversation away from inner experiences and toward more mundane subjects may assist in bringing the participant's awareness back to external reality. Simple motor acts such as taking a walk may also help with a participant's return to ordinary consciousness.

Expressive arts experiences can be powerful vehicles for self-exploration, self-awareness, and change. As such, they demand that we develop ourselves fully as artists, therapists, and human beings. To practice authentically, we must live with awareness of our own creative process as well as that of our clients. Expressive arts call us continually to hone our ability to enter into deeply sacred space and emerge to make manifest and give form to the wisdom found there. It is only through intimate knowledge of this process that we are prepared to facilitate the process for others.

SOLO VOICE
Becoming an Artist-Therapist

My life work for nearly thirty years now has been that of a teacher and a therapist. The practice of teaching and the practice of therapy are, for me, essentially about the same thing—creating a space in which we can grow as human beings, a space in which our individual uniqueness is recognized and our best potential is evoked. I seek to cultivate in my students, my clients, and myself the capacity to think in new and different ways about important ideas, ourselves, and our work. I want us to reflect deeply about what it means to be a human being within the larger historical, political, and cultural contexts in which we live. The kind of learning I seek is not just about acquiring information or finding answers. It is more about deepening the questions we are living: Who am I? What is the meaning of my life? How am I to live—in relationship to other human beings, in relationship to the natural world, and in relationship to whatever I believe is larger than my little self?

I was trained as a behavioral scientist and licensed to practice psychology, but I believe that the work I do and the life I live are more about art than science, although at the deepest level I don't see science and art as oppositional. The most meaningful learnings of my life have come from bearing witness to literally hundreds of human stories and from participating in our individual and collective creative experiences as the artists of our lives. To claim myself as an expressive therapist and teacher, as the artist of my own life, requires commitment to personal creative expression, to self-knowledge, and to daily practice. My life as an artist-therapist is nurtured within communities where trust, openness, integrity, passion, discipline, and mutual care and respect prevail. I am deeply committed to teaching and to living these values.

Working in the arts—writing, dancing, drumming, singing, performing rituals, and writing poetry—takes me to a deeper place than anything else I know. Poetry, especially, is the place where I can find the voice of my inner authority, a place where I can glimpse the truth I did not know I knew as in the following poem.

What the Artist Taught Me
(For Those Who Now Know)

When you can make art, you must
When you can't, you read
and watch TV.

Art goes with fine chocolate, champagne
and Wagner.
Art seeps into all your crevices
like a slow, soft river
Or crashes through your blood
like whitewater.

Art is alive.
It grabs you at night, keeps you
working until dawn,
In the morning keeps you
looking, looking
seeing with your whole body,
Keeps you open like flowers
bursting like seed pods,
Keeps you speaking aloud
The truth you did not know
you knew.

The work of therapy is about storytelling and story receiving, often reading between the lines to find the deepest meaning of the story. The privilege of bearing witness to story is one I do not take lightly. "Tell me, She Said" is a poem about that privilege.

Tell Me, She Said

Tell me, she said:
What is the story you are telling?
What wild song is singing itself through you?

Listen:
In the silence between there is music;
In the spaces between there is story.

It is the song you are living now.
It is the story of the place where you are.
It contains the shapes of these old mountains
The green of the rhododendron leaves,
It is happening right now in your breath,
In your heartbeat still drumming the deeper rhythm
Beneath your cracking words.

It matters what you did this morning and last
Saturday night and last year,
Not because you are important
But because you are in it and it is still moving,
We are all in this story together.

Listen:
In the silence between there is music;
In the spaces between there is story.

Pay attention:
We are listening each other into being.

"The Bone Hunters" reflects the work of therapy as the archaeology of story. We are looking for the essence, the ancient bone, that will tell us how our individual human stories are connected to the larger universal story of life.

The Bone Hunters

We are the bone hunters of the mind.
Dry-mouthed, we search the valleys of the soul,
Sift slowly, carefully, with reverence
Through the dust of eons,
Search for those pure relics,
Bleached white by a thousand suns,
The links that will connect us all,
The bone that speaks in a voice
Of reason to our small linear minds,
The bone seen by a single eye,
Which seeing one side only,
Still yearns to know at once
The many-sided human miracle,
All the facets of the turning stone.
We seek the bare bleached bones
Of human essence,
The heart's song,
The meaning of it all,
That we should each play out
These ancient stories
Told to children.
Of our children.

"Chaos Theory" and its accompanying watercolor/calligraphy collage "Deepest Impulse" (see cover art) are expressive of my personal philosophy of life and my experience of reality. It is also reflective of my personal work to integrate the scientist with the artist, to integrate rational and intellectual knowledge with body wisdom and intuitive and emotional knowing, to integrate ordinary life with mystical experience. Our objectivist epistemologies no longer suffice, and we reach forward and backward to remember who we are. New paradigms from biological and sociological systems theory, creativity theories, and quantum physics affirm our personal experience of the relational nature of reality. This poem and the collage reflect this view of reality.

Chaos Theory

We are living
in the in between
still reaching
to remember
our circles
of belonging.

There are so
many layers
of our little lives.
See how everything
falls away
into something larger.

In the quickening
gyre we see
the dark ones.
These are not monsters
but just the shapes
things want to come in.

The world is
not falling apart.
In the presence
of the quivering stars
our deepest impulse
is to dance.

The times in which we live, the rapid pace of life, the explosion of information, the expansion of technology, and the destruction of the natural environment are real aspects of a world that is both exciting and disturbing. We are living in chaos. Art making, living poiesis, is the only thing that makes any sense as a way of trusting in a larger and multidimensional whole.

—Sally Atkins

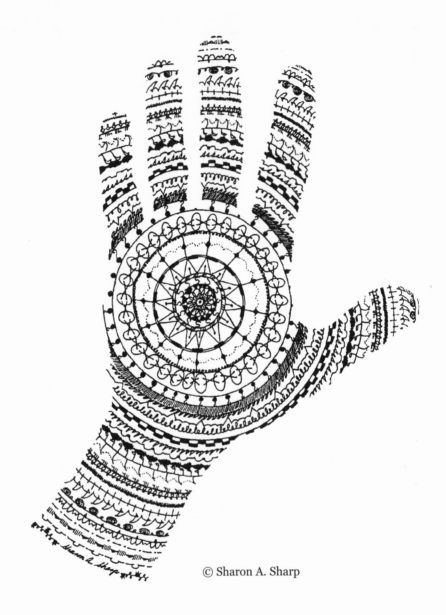

© Sharon A. Sharp

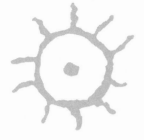

Part 2

CYCLES OF
CREATIVE PROCESS

*O*ur world cycles. There are cycles of life and death, seasonal cycles, cycles of the moon, cycles of day and night, cycles of inbreath and outbreath. In each of these cycles, there is rhythm in the waxing and waning, whether of the flowers, the moon, or the daylight. In each there is a time of emergence, a time of full outer manifestation, a time of fading that moves into a time of apparent dormancy when the activity is out of view. The paradox of cycles is that the apparent end is in reality the beginning of the next cycle. One is always linked to the next beginning.

So it is with the creative process. In creative expression, there is a period of beginning when the foundation is laid for the work that is to come, when the body and mind are prepared to enter into sacred space, when we open ourselves to listen with awareness for inspiration. Moving across the threshold requires that we let go of control, trusting that what is needed will be provided. As we move into the depths of the creative space, we may experience wonder, mystery, chaos, and emotions beyond anything we expect. In this ineffable space, we taste shadows, touch light, hear colors, smell memories. Often there is a gift, although it is rarely one we expect. As we emerge from the depths, we may struggle to name the experience, to find courage and voice to stand to the truth of who we are. As we claim our deepest wisdom, we bring the gift back to our lives, to our communities. As we integrate the newfound truth into our lives, we simultaneously prepare to enter the cycle again.

In creative expression, this cycle occurs on many levels at once. This cyclical pattern occurs in a single session, in a series of sessions, and in a lifetime of sessions. We are always in the cycle, even in times of apparent dormancy. It is important that we, as expressive arts therapists, honor the cycle of the client or group with whom we work.

The following chapters have been organized according to the cycles just described. Each of the chapters includes an overview, experiences appropriate for that cycle, personal stories, and poems related to that cycle. We invite you to enter into these cycles with us, with intention and awareness.

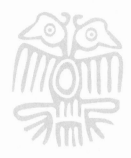

Chapter 3

BEGINNING

Daily Practice
We never get it right
It's life work
It has to do with being
Comfortably Alone

Honoring our interior lives
And finding our place in the larger world.
—Marianne Adams

*I*n order to move forward, within the cycle of creative expression, it is often necessary first to move backward. In order to jump, we must first squat down. In order to throw a ball, the hand first must go back. In order to shoot an arrow forward, we first must pull back on the string. To begin an action, it is often part of the beginning that we go in the opposite direction of the intended action. In the beginning, we expressive artists may need to discover our windup, our opposing motion that will help us release our creation. Each of us must find and know the center from which our inspirations come.

Daily practice is the beginning that becomes the ongoing participation in soul work. The ability to become and remain centered grows out of daily practice; the two are inseparable. As therapists, we must be able to draw upon our daily practice during our sessions so that we can be present and centered for our clients. Daily practice also allows for the renewal and focus necessary for staying in touch with our true selves. We must prepare a sacred space and then enter into that sacred space, removing all extraverted thoughts and images. Staying focused during the daily practice is a challenge, and being judgmental about this aspect of our practice can be damaging to the process itself.

Another element that is common to any type of daily practice is mindfulness— the ability to hold the present moment in awareness, to learn from it, and to release our preoccupation with the past or future. It is from the daily practice of mindfulness that we discover who we really are. Just about any repetitive activity in our lives can become a useful and revealing daily practice if we pay attention to the gifts that come from mindfulness. Over time, daily practice becomes a source of nourishment, a place of retreat, and a time to recognize the fabric of our interior lives.

The form of daily practice is highly individual; for some it may be painting one day and writing the next. Others may find they need to set a time and type of ritual in order to develop and maintain a habit of daily practice. For some, it may be as short as reading a meditation every morning over coffee. Others may find it helpful to engage a friend to establish a daily ritual such as walking. Each of us has the capacity to create sacred space, which becomes our container for growth, for our visions, our deepest wishes and our self-defined quests. This chapter presents exercises for opening to inspiration, examples of daily practice, and thoughts on the creative process.

Wellspring.
Source of energy,
Fountain of light.
Dancing, bubbling, rising deep within.
Bursts forth when contact is made.

—*Cathy McKinney*

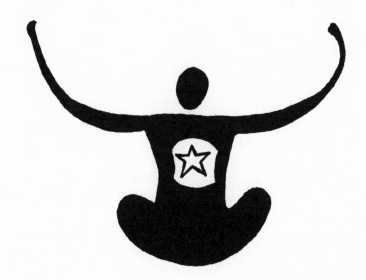

Opening to Inspiration

*In-spi-ra-tion: 1. the act of breathing in. 2. a divine influence
believed to qualify one to communicate sacred revelation.*

—Merriam-Webster's *Collegiate Dictionary*, 10th ed.

We open ourselves to inspiration in many ways. What follows
are some of the experiences we have found central in our own
creative endeavors. These experiences often serve as brief
transitions when we are moving from the outside world to the
inside. They also help us open the window to the inspiration
necessary for beginning the artistic endeavor. This list is not in any
way intended to be exhaustive. You will discover other sources in
your own experience. Experiment with these and others, and
become aware of sources that are always there for you.

Walks. Walking is universal; it is often an overlooked
pleasure of daily human experience. For some, the path may
involve long walks with old dogs and intimate friends. For others,
it may entail short, brisk walks to clear the brain. When we use
walking as a basis for inspiration, the emphasis shifts from exercise
to the soothing, calming effects of having a daily ritual. This
practice functions like a clearinghouse for letting the day's clutter
go. The constancy of walking the same walk daily becomes an
inspiration for spiritual growth, which in turn opens and deepens
one's artistic capacity.

Getting Sweaty. In addition to the proven physiological
benefits, getting sweaty seems to open our senses and release
tension that can keep us from receiving creative inspiration.
Getting sweaty often takes a fair amount of focus that can get us
beyond the point of self-consciousness. It is hard to be inhibited
and sweaty at the same time.

Rest. Perhaps the most overlooked source of inspiration for
many of us is rest. While a solid good night's sleep might be
optimal, the hectic pace of our lives may necessitate other options.
Creative solutions such as catnaps or even brief moments with our
eyes closed can refresh us, clear our thinking, and make us more
receptive to creative images and possibilities.

Listening. Quiet allows us the capacity to hear the music
that surrounds us—the birds chirping, the hum of the refrigerator,
the sound of the breeze, the rhythm and tempo of the machines in
our world. Listening absentmindedly to a wide variety of music, as

well as listening at other times with conscious intent, can stretch and inspire us.

Incubation. Sometimes inspiration comes from having the trust to allow an idea to lie fallow and attend to the mysterious glimpses that seem to come when we are not trying to work actively. It comes from paying attention to disparate images, movements, words, and emotions that have no apparent relationship to one another. There is no place for editorial censorship in this phase. Incubation does not care how long it takes to come to fruition.

Percolation. When a central idea has emerged, raw and formless, it is our job to allow and observe the wild, tender tendrils that shoot out from the central idea without trying to tame them or force them into shape. When they are ready, they will connect and order themselves. Our task is to maintain detached awareness. We are only the channels and witnesses for the process.

Others. Other people in our lives may serve as sources of creative inspiration. A word, a gesture, or a hug can serve as the vehicle for divine influence, for the bodily shift that leads us into creative space.

EXPLORATION
Tea Ceremony

In Japan, one beautiful tradition involves the tea ceremony. Although highly ritualized and elaborate, it is possible to bring some part of it into our lives for the purpose of centering. Find a quiet space surrounded by inspiring objects. Boil water in a teakettle, and meditate on the fire for heating the water as a metaphor for transforming energy. Pour the water slowly from the kettle into a special cup, as you listen to the sound the water makes. Finally, hold the cup in your hands, sit and drink the tea, and feel the nourishing heat through your body. Bask in the delicious silence.

EXPLORATION
Song Messages

The Gestalt therapist Barry Stevens (1969) advocates paying attention to the music we sometimes find playing "in our heads" for their messages. When you notice a tune "in your head," see if you can identify the title. Notice especially the lyrics that go with the phrase you hear. What is its message for you? What comment is it making on your present state? What is it calling you to do?

Centering

Even in the midst of chaos
There is a small, still center
Of absolute quiet,
Like the eye of a hurricane.

If I can find that center,
I can place myself within that stillness
And watch the world whirl by
In all of its beauty and agony.

And when, with clarity and serenity,
I can witness this spectacle
Some voice inside of me says:
"Yes, I see."

At last I can be fully present
To what is before me.
At last I can fully honor the unfolding
Of this desperate dance called "life."

—Terri Chester

Breathing as Daily Practice

We breathe. Hundreds of times an hour, thousands of times a day, we breathe. Usually our breathing is automatic, taken for granted. Most of the time, we attend to it only if it presents a challenge such as limitations due to illness or being "out of breath" from exertion. However, if we are attentive, it can both teach us and lead us toward wholeness.

On a biological level, the breath both brings oxygen necessary for survival and carries away carbon dioxide, the gaseous waste product of metabolism. Metaphorically, this action may also be seen as the continual process of bringing what is needed and carrying away what is no longer needed. In fact, the breath can carry much more than oxygen and carbon dioxide. It can cleanse us of tension, fatigue, pain, anxiety, and worry. It can bring calm, energy, peace, clarity, and stillness. The power to access the breath in this way is always there. We need only to allow it.

The breath can also carry our attention inward. It can take each of us to our center, to that sacred point from which inspiration arises. When we are at the center of our being, we may experience the stillness in the eye of the storm. From the center of our being, we may move out in new directions, into new dimensions, toward a deeper awareness of who we truly are. In the center, we may find ourselves connected with the source of our inspiration, with that which has been called the "seat of the soul" (Zukav, 1989). In that space, we have the opportunity to listen, receive, be refreshed, and be inspired.

SOLO VOICE
Daily Rituals

In the cultures of indigenous peoples all over the world, rituals of song, dance, drama, and storytelling mark the passages of life and carry the cultural teachings about how to live. In our culture many of us hold to religious rituals of baptism, marriage, and funeral rites, but many aspects of ritual as a part of daily personal life and family life are lost to us. For some, the common rituals of daily life are watching television or shopping at the mall. Unless we are gardeners, even our place in the turning of daily, monthly, and seasonal cycles of the natural world may be lost to us.

Ritual is marked by intention, focus, and meaning. Something in us hungers for ritual. We borrow the rituals of other countries—drumming from West Africa, vision quests and sweat lodge ceremonies of the Native Americans, and solstice rituals from the ancient Celts.

Small personal rituals have become a valuable part of my own daily practice:

Morning Cleansing

I splash cold water on my face—four rounds to honor the directions and the elements in which I live, of which I am made:

East—the place of vision, new beginnings, spring, air
South—the place of innocence, full flowering, summer, fire
West—the place of introspection, death and transformation, autumn, water
North—the place of wisdom, dormancy, winter, earth

Focusing

I read a meditation, poem, or quote, or allow a thought to enter and deepen my intention, my experience of the day. I take time to reflect.

Pouring Warmth

After the family has eaten and left for work and school, I pour a sacrament of coffee and milk. I hold the cup, warm in my hand. I take the time to smell, taste. Just that.

Writing as Prayer

I light a candle for writing. I honor the light, the lifeforce, and I open to receive what may come. I give up trying to do something, to say something. The empty page becomes my container. I watch and feel the flow of ink on the page, enjoying the pleasure of the slowness of my calligraphic pen, the pleasure of sometimes beautiful letters. This way I must slow down. I seek the one clear word to catch the meaning. It is a discipline of precision, of claiming space and time.

—*Sally Atkins*

Poetry as Daily Practice

Daily practice is fundamental to my life as an artist. My primary practices, in addition to walking, are a practice of personal body prayer, based on a twenty-five-year practice of yoga, and writing. I have kept a personal journal since I was nine. Recently I have been practicing calligraphy as a part of my daily writing practice in order to slow down, to experience my writing as a form of meditation. "Writing Ritual" illustrates the magic of this practice for me.

Writing Ritual

Some days
Everyone who walks
Into your stare is beautiful,
The old Black man
In his leather cap
On the corner of Coxe Avenue
And Haywood Street,
The pale waiter
In the basement café.

I won't argue magic anymore
All I have
Is just this ritual now,
Writing,
Drinking coffee, listening
To an old Bob Dylan song.

—*Sally Atkins*

EXPLORATION
Personal Rituals

Think carefully about the ordinary personal rituals in your life. Which of your daily habits could become a ritual for you? How would your attention shift to make this practice a more intentional part of your life? Write or draw about a ritual experience in your life.

SOLO VOICE
Daily Practice for Spiritual and
Personal Growth

I like using the expression "daily practice" to imply the routine or consistency, to describe the ordinariness and fundamental nature of the beast. In truth, I do not have a daily practice. I actually have four practices: writing, walking (hiking in the summer), yoga, and a gratitude ritual. I do one of these almost every day of my life. Over the years, these practices, which started as recreation or hobbies, have become the foundation that stabilizes my life and feeds my creative process. Strange to think that a structure or routine that grounds my life could also be a source of creative energy. I used to think of routine and discipline as being constraining and confining. Now I find the ritual of these practices soothing and nurturing. Sinking into the familiar rhythms of these activities is part of what allows me to access that deep connection to the source of my creativity—indeed, the source of my life.

I have been writing the longest, and of the four practices, writing is most essential to my process and my life. Several years ago, I bought Natalie Goldberg's book Writing Down the Bones (1986). Later I bought her second book, Wild Mind: Living the Writer's Life (1990). I have to give her credit for planting the seed of the idea that writing is a discipline, that indeed it can become a daily practice for spiritual growth. Since reading her books, I have been using writing in a more intentional way—not just as a coping skill but as a vehicle for personal growth and development. I also found the "morning pages" process described in Julia Cameron's The Artist's Way (1992) useful and inspiring. Although I don't always write every day, I write most days. And the way I approach my writing is different now. I sit down at the paper and see what comes.

Walking is a practice that also grew from a love and started as a sort of recreational activity. I have always loved being outside and walking or hiking. And as with writing, over time the walking has developed a spiritual aspect. I have taken many "pilgrimages" around my local area in search of clarity or comfort or solitude.

I have been studying for five years with a wonderful teacher who has been instructing me on how to use yoga to become more healthful and comfortable not only in my body but in my life. And although it is a newer addition to my life, yoga is the practice that has taken me more deeply into my writing, walking, work, homelife, and other areas.

Recently, I added a ritual based on Sarah Breathnach's Simple Abundance (1995). Every night in bed before I turn out the light I make a gratitude list, which includes every thing, person, or experience that I feel grateful for. It may be, for example, a conversation I had with someone, the weather, a good meal I ate, or a book I read. After only six months, I am already reaping the benefits of this acknowledgment of my abundance. There have been several nights after difficult or frustrating or painful days when I went to bed feeling overwhelmed but gained some perspective and balance by listing all of the things I was grateful for.

Actually, one of the wonderful things about a having daily practice is that it does transfer to other areas of life—even the seemingly unrelated areas. Over time, I have become conditioned by my practices. I begin to relax almost immediately upon stepping into the yoga space. Even now as I write about that experience I take a deep breath, relax my shoulders, stretch my neck...and soon begin to notice what it takes to re-create that experience in other areas of my life. And there are other benefits. I am learning that sometimes it is enough to just show up at yoga class, sit down with my journal, or put on my hiking boots. As soon as I begin the ritual, the rhythms take over and I can do what needs to be done.

Through my practices, I've learned that it is okay to just start somewhere to prime the pump. It is okay to just do a rough draft of the paper, the project, the conversation, the errand. I am learning to pay attention and to focus. I am learning to become my own container, instead of using external resources (situations or people) to hold my life. I am learning how to listen to my body, to my intuition, sometimes to the conflict between my head and heart. I am learning to use my daily practices as a tool to dig out those needs and dreams and create a space for what I most value.

—*Terri Chester*

Yoga Embrace

Welcome, says the floor.
I am here to give you my hardnesss
so you may know the shape
of your bones. Yes, says the air,
I offer my fullness to surround
you with support and teach you
the flow, in and then out.
Here, say the birds, the bugs, the
rustling leaves, the rain, the voices—
we sing the song that pulses
through your veins, that lets
your mind knowingly relax
to take it all in and feel
your breath, feel your rhythm,
enjoy your skin, and drink in this
rich goodness of today.

—Sharon A. Sharp

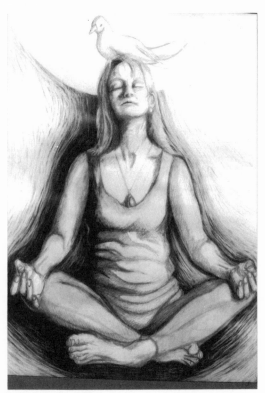

© Lori Fowler-Hill

SOLO VOICE
Discovery in Dance

In its essence, dance teaches a person to be present and to attend to the sensation of the moment. The practice of taking a daily class becomes a reminder to focus intention, a continuous process of working more deeply for clarity, rhythm, and expression. The fact that class is often a communal practice gives support for the discipline that is needed to humble ourselves daily to go through the opening process again and again and again. The fact that there are generally no sick days, paid leaves, or retirement plans adds to the intensity of being present in the experience in dance.

As a part of most dancers' lives there is a strict, devoted adherence to the necessity of taking a daily technique class; it is generally accepted as a sacrosanct ritual. About twenty years ago, I began the daily ritual of doing a ballet barre, alone, when I did not have access to taking a class. Initially, it was a way of nourishing and taking care of myself and provided much-needed alone time. Often, it became the initial impetus for creative work. Ultimately, my solitary practice began to lose its internal focus; facing my faults in the mirror began to seem too much like a daily confessional.

Gradually, over time my attitude about daily class changed, and I wasn't sure why. Perhaps it was being out of the routine of taking daily class, or my age, or my perspective, but I had a hard time taking class or my practice seriously. Since I was unsure of how to start over for myself, I spent some time feeling guilty about my lack of discipline and motivation; I was a little lost. At this point in my life, I needed a daily practice that would go beyond the physical. My needs were deeper than high extensions, technical speed, and triple turns. I was looking for growth that was more multidimensional, more internally focused, plus something that would feed my creative energies.

I was drawn to explore Joseph Pilates's (Siler, 2000) body–mind method for its claims of increased mindfulness, strengthening, and flexibility. Pilates originally called his method Contrology, which he defined as the "complete coordination of body, mind, and soul" (Pilates, quoted in Pilates and Miller, 1998). Pilates developed his approach to unify the Western emphasis on physical activity and the Eastern emphasis on mental concentration. The Pilates method uses more than five hundred exercises. Floor exercises are often taught in group mat classes, but the method is generally taught one on one, using several different pieces of equipment that Pilates originally began developing in the 1920s.

I was particularly interested in this method as it enhanced physical conditioning, precision of movement, proper breathing, and release. The focus is internal, stressing centered, balanced, and attentive movement. Again and again, economical effort and precision of movement are presented as ideals. Breath is the impetus for any effort. Claims of injury rehabilitation and neutralizing of muscular imbalances appealed to me due to the chronic hip tendinitis I was experiencing.

I was also intrigued with the Pilates claim of establishing very strong and lengthened muscles. Now after deeper study, I am impressed by how it has affected not only the way I dance but my ability to be centered, attentive, and present in my body. I am more able to feel movement from internal sensation, as opposed to taking external visual cues from the mirror. I also work more from the central core of my body, rather than by sheer muscle and willpower, allowing for more three-dimensional freedom and ease in my movement. I have begun to appreciate the Zen-like qualities of the Pilates method. For me, daily practice of the Pilates method feels like a moving meditation. From consistent, inwardly directed practice, my joy in dancing has become available and visible once again. It has been my vehicle for learning to move *not by my effort*.

I have also established a new daily ritual for myself that could keep me teaching and dancing for the next twenty-plus years. I have replaced my waning old habit of taking daily technique class with one that suits my current needs much more; the Pilates work is solitary, thorough, and, to me at age forty-plus, gratifying on physical and spiritual levels.

—Marianne Adams

Dancing can be anything
(Lessons from David Dorfman)

I've always thought, or perhaps been taught,
That dancing was for the tall and small boned or the
petite and breastless
Not for the ordinarily shaped or unusually proportioned
Most definitely not for the medium and thick
Who save what little grace we possess for lay-ups and
digs.

Dancing is not like that
Dancing can be anything
Dancing does not have to be relegated
To the secrecy of living rooms, bedrooms, or secret places
Dancing is one of those places that talks without words
Dancing can be anything.

—Jill Masten-Byers

SOLO VOICE
Mysteries of Creative Process

Often, the creative process comes to life when being creative is allowed, honored, valued. Sometimes this comes out of necessity or by nurturing or by fumbling or stumbling along. Recently, I watched my old sheepdog tire herself while looking frantically around the house to find a place to bury a huge rawhide bone. Of course, she wanted to go outside for a proper burial of her treasure, but due to the weather, I was reluctant to let her out.

I felt as if I were witnessing her creative process take over when she began to shift and work within the constraints and limitations I had superimposed. She burrowed into the corner of a closet and deliberately began her work, rooting and digging, pushing and pawing shoes, shirts, and yarn into a camouflage grave for her precious bone. She had gone from indecision and fretting into action. It was focused, nonjudgmental, resplendent work. Panting, lunging, and nosing, she was fully engaged in a creative, brilliant, imperfect solution. Her pleasure in this experimental creative act was evident. I can think of no better illustration of the mystery of the creative process.

As I begin to contemplate the mystery of creative process, I find myself wandering, searching, looking for clues, feeling uneasy, looking for space, wishing to find time for the elusive muse called creativity to appear. How do I begin my own creative process? Is that knowledge ever visible? Can anyone really explain a process that is so amorphous? How and where I start comes out of who I am, the sum of my experiences and my current frame of reference. Am I feeling easy and open, receptive to what is? Or is my life feeling cluttered and uncentered? Most often it is some mixture in between. Maddeningly incongruent, I float, fall, soar, and sink.

For me, creative images and awarenesses generally come as unsought, unplanned insights. These moments of receptivity are often surprising, coming as I am trying to e-mail someone about something totally unrelated or cooking dinner. It is a place of unattachment, of wonder, of discovery, of deep mystery. It is a place of relaxed attention. At that moment, my creative process begins to flow. Just like the yeast that is integral to bread making, the creative process bubbles, smells, dies back, and eventually disappears into bread, but it is the substance that is behind the rising. Both are elements of transformation.

Space unfolds when I am away from others (or after a good laugh) or have spoken my heart with an intimate friend. Sometimes it happens in the night, when I awake with an image and have the presence to follow it into movement or jot it in a journal. Often I must physically make the space for myself by closing a door, taking a bath, putting on headphones, or dozing in a catnap. Sometimes it comes as I literally clear away clutter from my life. Filing papers (however absurdly), cleaning off my desk, and ordering my space all become part of my preparatory process. Because my conscious mind is focused on the task at hand, my creative self is free to begin, without the editor, the critic, the expectant demon who always wants a perfect product. Rules begin to bend, blur, and dissolve as I begin to trust my circuitous and unimaginable process.

Time comes less easily; distractions abound. Why is it always so much easier to tackle a much less meaningful task? There are many more reasons not to do this work than I can think of to do it, but none is as powerful as the need to create, the need to know myself and understand the world through my own art making.

Paradoxically, it is the time when I know myself the most clearly and I am the least familiar to myself.

It seems that the pain and pleasure of being lost and finding our way and the complexity that allows us to hold both are inherent in this thing called creative process. Part of the mystery is why fear recedes long enough for us to create and how time can stretch and zoom and feel circular all at the same time. How safe, magical, and elastic time and space can feel when we are in the midst of our own creative process.

In this place, we do not step back to ask why; we are instinctual. We move as with guidance, or spiritual blessings. It is as if we are being led by our hearts to our deeper wisdom, our unconscious knowing. In this moment we are connected to our most hidden truths and linked to the knowledge of the oceans and the earth and to our spirit ancestors. These mysteries of the creative process appear when we let go of expectations (of where bones should be buried) and give in to the implausible!

—Marianne Adams

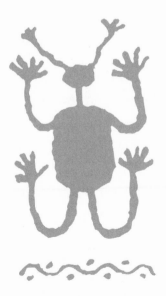

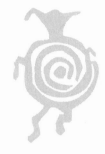

Chapter 4

MOVING INWARD

Awakening

Into the mug of morning
pour yourself, warm
and dark, your aromatic
presence hugging the hand-
formed divide between
inside and out. Ease
from empty into full
until, brim-level, you
rise and swirl, a steamy
mist rejoining its source.

—Sharon A. Sharp

$\mathcal{M}$oving inward is a moment within the cycle where the threshold of trust is approached. It is vital to trust in your body, your self, and your ability. This is often the place where the judgmental inside voice is first encountered during the creative process: "You are not ready. You don't have the skills. You will make a fool of yourself. It is easier not to do this. You are not an artist." As soon as you hear this voice, it is important to take a moment and consciously dialogue with it, to gently tell it that you need its support, and to imagine joining with this interior part of yourself and walking together through the threshold to the inside. Once this dialogue is established, it may be necessary to continue the dialogue throughout the entire cycle. It is helpful to recognize that everyone has this doubting voice inside and that all artists and creators find ways of accepting and working with this part of themselves. Transforming this voice in a positive and playful way can be more productive than attempting to fight it. Images such as singing a duet or dancing a pas de deux may be helpful.

Once trust is firmly grounded and a working relationship with the inner voice is established, moving inward becomes fluid. The feeling is that of delightful anticipation, as opposed to tentative fear. It is the difference between running and jumping into the ocean instead of sticking in your big toe and thinking, "I don't know about this—there are things in the water that I can't see, and the water is really cold!" The beauty of trusting your ability to move inward is that whether or not the muses are there to greet you, the ability to knock on the door and enter is always present.

This chapter presents poems, essays, and experiences for moving inward. They are meant to inspire, provide thoughtful insight, and present concrete ways for entering inside. They are a playground for developing the necessary trust and confidence to cross the threshold into exploring ourselves through art.

SOLO VOICE
Motion

We are told by physicists that everything is in motion: The entire cosmos—including the planet we live on, the molecular structure of our bodies, and even the most solid-seeming stone—when internally understood, is a universe of space and motion. To paraphrase a conversation I once had with the noted music therapist Charles Eagle, "If it isn't in motion, it doesn't exist."

We are beings in and of motion, yet we find ourselves saying words like, "When my life settles down a bit, I'll be okay." Of course, efforts to counter what may seem like a life of chaos with some sense of order and simplicity may prove fruitful. We have received many spiritual commandments such as "Be still and know that I am God," but I dare say that even if we could become still, the God we would come to know would be in motion. It may also be that in order to find true stillness, we must first connect with our internal motion.

I believe that to understand and live the lives that we would most like to live, we must come to terms with knowing and becoming comfortable with our motion, both internal and external. It has been noted that even a piece of furniture exists first as thought, is described with drawings and dimensions, and is manifest as a spinning mass of molecules. Even then, it is on its way to returning to the earth from which it came as decaying pieces of fabric and wood breaking down into simpler carbon structures. It has been noted, too, that everything is becoming something else. Children are becoming young adults, coal is becoming diamond, leaves fall from trees and decay, and so on. How we choose to acknowledge and consciously connect with what we are becoming and what we have set in motion may be important if only because it pulls us away from thinking of ourselves as finished products. We think, "I am a father, worker, husband, brother, driver, musician, and so on." Even further, we define and judge ourselves as, "I am a good, bad, excellent, superb, or poor this, that, or the other."

Having so defined myself with various descriptions and roles, I can now separate myself from the fear of what it feels like to be in motion. What could be scarier than having been flung through space? What could seem less controlled than to acknowledge that all we create has motion of its own, which may or may not fit our conscious imprint? Conversely, what could be more exciting than this kind of ride and this kind of evolving creation? Our choice is evident: learn to move in faith or futilely try to get a grip on life. The latter would be like trying to grab and hold onto light.

—*Harold McKinney*

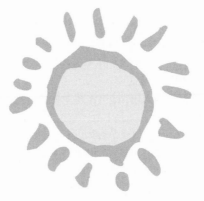

Wrightsville Beach

Betwixt the dunes
*   and the lick of turquoise*
Lay the old souls
Crushed by the current   *Wash over me*
Abraded by the undertow   *Wash over me*
Polished by the waves   *Wash over me*
Yielding to the power
*   larger than themselves.*

No pity, no sorrow,
Peace lives here.
Joy resides here.
Their essence shines here.

—Kate Brinko

EXPLORATION
The Point of Stillness

We have been created to move and to set our own creations in motion. Florice Tanner gave the following exercise in the book *Basic Energies in Wholeness*. Tanner subtitles this exercise as "the still point where inner becomes outer and outer becomes inner" (p. 61). Try using the exercise as a prelude to sculpting, painting, drawing, composing, dancing, performing, or connecting to the motion of a piece of music through listening. The altered state of consciousness afforded by the exercise may move us closer to "reality" than do our illusions of solidity. It also may provide us with some fluidity with which to experience creation. Read one paragraph of the exercise at a time and take a few moments at the end of each to close your eyes and be fully aware of the sensations in your body.

We have built-in equipment for holistic functioning. It is normal in response to an idea to exhale and release an energy charge, relaxing the body downward simultaneously with releasing the active timing element of the energy charge upwards. Such a balanced habit of release gives a readiness set for whatever follows. Any restriction causes negative stresses.

Sit comfortably with your feet on the floor and your hands resting comfortably on your knees. Sway from side to side comfortably. Close your eyes. Gradually diminish the outer swaying until there is no visible physical movement, but continue the inner sensation of swaying. Gradually diminish this inner awareness of swaying until it reaches a point. Try to locate this point, or center, exactly. Determine if this point is static or ever changing slightly.

❀

Continue the sensation of swaying, ever so slightly, at the point in your breathing center. Then direct your thought to the central arch [in the palm of] one hand as it rests on your knee. Do not outwardly move your hand but imagine lifting it. Can you feel a relationship between the center arch in your hand and your breathing center? If not, try again until you succeed.

❀

Then try the other hand.

❀

Imagine lifting your foot from its sensitive arch.

❀

Repeat these experiments until you sense a connection between your breathing center and the sensitive centers in your hands and feet.

❀

Sense a relationship between the point in your breathing center and your periphery. Try now to establish a definite sensation between your breathing center and the circumference of your room, your community, your state, and your friend.

❀

At your own pace, move now to the arts experience of your choice.

Refuge

Feeling flat, plain,
torn, bare, I seek
the blank peace of paper,
the dark flow of ink so
I can draw out the core
of my fiber, unfold
the dreamworld stretching
beyond margins, move
from edge to edge not
feeling cornered. Through
lines, letters, and scribbles
I hear my voice without speaking,
tell my truths and my lies
that lead to truths as they
take shape, no erasing,
no redoing. Then the flat,
plain, torn paper bears
witness to the fullness
of my silences and the depths
of my surface explorations.

—*Sharon A. Sharp*

SOLO VOICE
Fear as a Gift

Fear informs. The sound of a rattlesnake strikes fear in the heart of a hiker, saving his life as he jumps away. A toddler stops at the edge of a precipice because of her fear of high places. A middle-aged man gives up smoking because of his fear of what he may be doing to his health. The gift of this kind of fear seems obvious.

But what about the irrational fears? The fear of speaking in public or phobias about flying, crowds, open spaces or closed spaces—these and a host of other paralyzing fears can also bring gifts of their own. They can give us information about who we are, where we have been wounded, and how we may want to direct our energy for personal growth and expansion.

Situations that cause fear vary widely. For a musician, it may be a particular performance situation. For an artist, it might be a certain kind of exposure for her work. For a criticized author, it might be the thought of starting a new book. For a teacher, it might be the risk of trying a certain approach to a class. Each of these may indicate to the frightened individual involved that this is fertile ground for his art. The classically trained musician who would really like to try to improvise but has not done so because of her fear of extending herself beyond the written notes may find that even the smallest baby steps in that direction bring new freedom to her overall musicianship, greater confidence to her classical performance, and even a new willingness to extend herself in her relationships.

I found myself dreading a particularly demanding musical performance in which I was to be involved. Every time I thought about what I had obligated myself to do, my heart raced and I felt the entire "fight or flight" response take over my body. Over the days and even weeks before the performance, I learned to stay with the fear each time it came. Instead of redirecting my thoughts to escape the fear, I decided to just let it have its way with me.

© Lori Fowler-Hill

As you might guess, each time my heart raced, I felt a rush of adrenaline; but I also discovered that my fear did not overpower me. I began to appreciate the courage I was developing with this response, courage that would not have been exercised had there been no fear to draw it out. I was beginning to understand M. C. Richards when she said, "Come my fear and sit with me and I will marry thee." Fears, once noted, can be celebrated as friends. They signal the edges of new growth and offer invaluable guidance.

-Harold McKinney

SOLO VOICE
Resistance

> *Resistance is like a holding tank.*
> *It still exists even if you choose not to look.*
> *Greet your resistance.*
> *Name your demons.*
> *They shape your journey*
> *In the sun as well as the night.*

The artist as an impostor, that is my usual distraction. The noise I can create to this score can be endless. Although the variations can go on ad nauseam, the refrain is this: "That's awful—how can you call yourself an artist? Maybe if I just fix it before anyone else sees it. Why can't you be a creative genius? If you were really smart, this would work...blah, blah, blah." (See Plate #2.)

All my noise has to do with judgment of my work, a form of taking myself out of the process and assigning value to the product. For me, resistance is part of my creative process. If I work through it, it allows me to deepen, to drop into a place beyond consciousness. From there, the journey takes me blindly. It is about having the mindfulness not to censor what does not make sense. It often leads me to a place where I don't think I am ready to go. And for me, that blind, uneven, unnavigable path is unavoidable if I choose to create from any type of self-knowledge or growing edge. I have never made a dance like the one I set out to make, regardless of what I may say at the time of creation. The meaning of a dance evolves and reveals itself over time.

—Marianne Adams

Fears

Fear of abandonment
>   Not physical but emotional
>   Permanent, not negotiable
Fear of the dark
>   Not of what's in the dark
>   But of the absence of light
Fear of being alone
>   Not for an evening or even a lifetime
>   But of a lifetime of empty conversation
>   A lifetime on an island where
>   No one speaks the language of my heart.

The Race

Sometimes it scares me
How well I deceive even myself
Now and then I catch glimpses of myself
In the looking glass
As I pass
At a dead run,
Caught up in my race
To find out who I am
And destroy the evidence
Before anyone else catches on.

—Terri Chester

Improvisation: Three Voices

Im-pro-vise: *1. To compose, or simultaneously compose and perform, on the spur of the moment and without any preparation; extemporize. 2. a) To bring about, make, or do on the spur of the moment. b) to make, or do, with the tools or materials at hand, usually to fill an unforeseen and immediate need [to make a bed out of leaves].*

—Webster's New World Dictionary

Openness to Possibilities: Marianne

At its best, improvisation is the time in the process when all possibilities are still open and there are no barriers of self-consciousness. In any improvisational experience, I swing primarily between two modes: one is joyful, giddy, humorous, and playful, and the other is fearful...fearful that I'll be exposed and nothing will be there. One place that I hold this fear physically is at the base of my skull and my cranial vertebrae. So when I work to find and free some cranial space, my visceral reaction is often to become dizzy and somewhat disoriented and, at the same time, to feel wildly, euphorically free. Other times, the reaction is not so physically apparent. It is about allowing the process despite fear, thus permitting myself to continue in scary places. For this reason, it is about allowing play and fear to coexist, staying connected, and being fully present. In any improvisation, there is always a search for connection and ways to integrate a deeper meaning into my work.

Surprise in the Music: Cathy

Solo improvisation is, for me, almost always at the piano; it flows out of feeling both emotion and the bodily "felt sense" described by Gendlin (1981) that accompanies the emotion. First comes a chord or a single tone, then another, then another, each showing the way to the next, each moving a little more deeply into feeling. As the music creates itself through me, it rejoices in the joy, penetrates and cradles the pain, or gives bombastic voice to the anger.

There is always a surprise in the music—in where it leads, in unexpected sonorities, in how it grows. But regardless of where it begins or ends, I am changed by the experience. The feeling shifts—sometimes becoming more present and focused, sometimes diminishing with the release that comes from being heard.

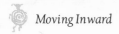

Falling into a Note: Harold

Improvisation must begin with an examination of the material with which to improvise, a note, a couple of notes, a scale, or a preexisting melody. Otherwise, there is just too much. One can't improvise with all of it (God's already doing that). My improvisation must come out of an absorption in some small something, in that moment when I fall into a note or a phrase and see where it leads.

Cold at the Poet's Fire

Where did it go
the kiss of flame
that once brought blood
to my lips?

I have been robbed
of my nights
when, like stars,
the muses danced their wild

spirits on my tongue
and blew kyrie eleisons
to wake the beauty
sleeping in me

Now they knit and pearl
their faces to the wall
as I beg at their door
with my empty bowl

I knock and wait
for a voice
to entice me
to the poet's fire

but the door is thick
with silence
and only snow
fills my bowl

—Kirtan Coan

SOLO VOICE
Falling through the Mouthpiece

As a performing musician, I was initially attracted to expressive arts work because of a desire to recapture in my own performance something of an experience I had had as a listener in the audience at a wonderful music recital in 1969. The performer had demonstrated naturalness in his approach to "singing" through his instrument, and that left me transformed. It seemed that a door to an infinite place of knowing opened during the music and I was overwhelmed with an indescribable confidence in the benevolence of the universe and all that moves within it to complete its perfect work in a way that would leave every being infinitely blessed.

Many years later I went to study with this performer and was given a dream that encompassed the essence of his teaching. In the dream I found myself falling through space through one trombone mouthpiece after another. While they seemed tiny at first, they provided plenty of space for my passage. The experience was quite frightening. Nevertheless, as I jettisoned my way through the throat of each mouthpiece and fell through one space to another, I began to get the feel of letting go and falling through the space provided. I woke in a cold sweat, thinking I must have been practicing too much.

However, the next day when I approached my practice, I knew in my body the meaning of the dream. The music I wished to produce could only be realized through a sense of accepting and letting go to the motion of the air that was being projected through the instrument. Before, I had been trying to release the music through the instrument while simultaneously attempting to control that which had been set in motion. This was similar to a golfer trying to push the ball to the hole with the club when the club could be used more beautifully, efficiently, and naturally when released to the forces of gravity and momentum. The vulnerability encountered in such an act resembled the fear in falling, but the freedom I gained in musical expression would not have been attainable otherwise.

Later, as a teacher in a music school, I found great joy in connecting with other artists, poets, dancers, and therapists who had discovered something of this access to artistic and personal freedom. Fellow explorers of the vulnerable shared with each other

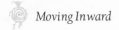

and each other's students their personal successes and failures in accessing such magic.

How does one do his part in originating artistic motion and still demonstrate how and when to get out of the way? How do I practice my art and live with mindfulness of my responsibility while also acknowledging my limitations for true accomplishment, which can be gained only by cooperation with natural law? What are the specifics of that law, and how may real accomplishment be accessed more consistently? I am still in the midst of exploring these questions, with a great sense of privilege at being involved with others who hold similar priorities.

—Harold McKinney

SOLO VOICE
Inviting Poetry

The Muses have usually been pictured as women since classical Greek times, perhaps because when the muse, say of poetry, is chased, she merely runs away; but when one prepares, waits, and attends, she will appear and nurture the supplicant by opening his or her senses and emotions—the receptors. So the beginning of poetry is preparing to receive. However, the act of poetry is the act of "kenning"—knowing in the sense of understanding from within, or loving in the fullest sense. That's not to say poetry is always soft and sweetly romantic; knowing isn't always approving or even liking. Anger is as appropriate to poetry as any other emotion, but it cannot be mere projection; it must come from knowing the focused-on individual or event intimately, and, to be genuine, the emotion must be "in spite of" the love one feels when possessed of intimate knowledge.

Thus, my most common starting place for poetry is observation. I'm an introverted and intuitive person with a tendency to miss details, so focused attention, especially when directed outwardly, is an altered state of consciousness for me; the world appears fresh, clear, and alluring to the imagination. I like to sit quietly outside and simply watch what is going on. But even that requires preparation.

I ask students to focus on their breath for about three minutes, then I give them a raisin or other piece of fruit and have them close their eyes, smell it, touch it, put the fruit in their mouths, roll it around, feel it, focus on it. Finally, I allow them to bite, and I ask that they follow the path of the sweet juice very carefully. Next, I have them open their eyes, trying to maintain the level of focus as they place it outside themselves, on whatever they experience. They may then move very, very slowly outdoors and touch, be aware of the temperature, their own feet on the pavement or ground, any individual spider, blade of grass, or event that calls their attention. (I learned this exercise from the parents of one of my students, Geoffrey Freeman.)

Fortunately, for my own work, I no longer have to use the piece of fruit; I've done it enough that I can slip into that attitude of consciousness just by being outside by myself. Focusing in that way never fails to draw me out of myself into a refreshing encounter and seldom fails to spark a poem for me.

The muse is often generous, acting out of grace, for I will sometimes simply hear a rhythm and begin writing to it, trusting that something worthwhile will happen. Occasionally, a line or two will spontaneously appear. The trick in that case, too, is to be prepared to receive whatever is coming. The beginning of poetry is receptivity, so if one thinks of oneself as a poet, the emergent words will take precedence. I've also tried to become receptive by listing all the significant people in my life and writing dialogues with them to see what emerges. Often the result is a poem. I've also listed the themes of my life and my interests. Not surprisingly, some themes have persisted for many years, so all I have to do is call up the theme and new ideas for poems appear. Dreams, fantasies, or odd words can all begin a poem if I'm ready, but I certainly don't just wait for inspiration; I prepare and invite. If the muse doesn't notice me, I can always revise and craft the raw poems waiting to be finished.

—Jay Wentworth

Apple Walk

Experience surprises me:
The moment's lacy intricacy
is not decoration but substance.
The chunk of apple admired
for its white meat and alluring skin
felt in slick and textured contrast
is not the stuff of metaphor
because so like itself alone. Heard,
the apple performs a ragged decrescendo
of chewing. Tasted, with eyes closed,
its cool juice dribbles over the tongue
exciting sweet spots until only
a vaguely bitter pulp remains.

Such awareness borne lightly
out-of-doors shines clearly
on peeking rhododendron pink
and the ancient work of ants and bees.
Whole new landscapes leap fresh
from familiar obscurity: A stream
is born, a tree full of finches; a puddle
on a barrel top is so real to my hand,
I feel my penis stir.

In deep enjoyment of this state,
I head for the library, carried
by feet that can distinguish cement
from asphalt and grass from dirt. Life
is everywhere, spiny defiance in a pit
of road or creatures clinging, running
along walls. The walls themselves
with a face or word on the odd brick.
The air is alive with perfumed fingers
every tree enflaming me with secret flowers.

I wake from this emergent world
many blocks beyond my destination.

—Jay Wentworth

EXPLORATION
Listening to the Body

Before You Begin: Read through this exercise once or twice before doing it on your own. Don't worry if you don't do it just as I have written; the parts you leave out are probably not important to you. Repetition of this exercise will allow you greater freedom to know and expand your own possibilities. In this experience, you are asked to discover new ways of stretching your body. You can prepare for this experience by breathing deeply for a few minutes. The structure for this experience is very simple: start standing, move all the way down to lying on the floor, and then rise to standing again. The main point is to follow your breath. If you feel stuck, just use this time to be still and breathe. If you stay with it, your breath will carry you until the next movement becomes apparent. Allow yourself about five minutes for each section; the whole experience will take approximately fifteen to twenty minutes.

To learn from this experience, you must trust in what your body whispers to you. Focus inward. You may want to start to listen with your eyes closed. You'll become aware of gurgles, tight spots, pleasurable moments, and resistance—each will give you clues about where to go next. Move at your own pace, which may differ from others'. Respect your own limitations, and trust and honor your particular safety needs, both emotionally and physically. There is no preset shape or plan of how your movement should look; you are simply asked to do what feels good, and indulge in the sensation of soothing, gradual, playful movement. It is optimal to have a quiet space and time for reflection afterward.

To Begin: Start by standing with your eyes closed and begin to sense the flow of movement that feels right to you. You can open your eyes anytime you need to. Try to move through all your joints, allowing yourself to experience an easy, continuous, downward motion. When you find a tight spot, allow yourself to spend some time with it. Can you discover a way to sense more freedom and ease in that area? Gradually move as slowly as you can toward the floor, reaching and elongating in ways that you have never consciously tried before. Try not to rely on stretches that you have done in the past, but instead try to explore new ways of sensing length. Allow yourself the freedom to experience new movement possibilities with ease. What does that feel like? Can you feel a release in different areas of your body at the same time? Can you allow yourself to feel more sensation in your spine?

Whenever you are stuck, just pay attention to your breath. If you can stay with the stillness and trust it, your breath will carry you until the next movement becomes apparent. Once you have made it to the floor, allow time to get comfortable on the floor; give yourself over to the floor. Can you allow yourself to spread, release, twist and curl, spiral, and roll? Paying attention to sensation allows you access to many body systems. The rhythms of your blood pulsing and heart beating, your breath, the fluidity of your organs, the language of your muscles and bones all offer clues about your internal state. Can you be completely absorbed in sensation? Can you focus internally enough to feel the pleasure of sequential movement throughout your spine? Be as indulgent and as slow moving as you dare!

As a transition, before moving up off the floor, allow yourself a moment of complete peaceful stillness. When you are ready, see if you can come to standing in a way you have never consciously done before. You might imagine yourself as a plant or an animal or a star—whatever gives you a sense of freedom and adventure. Or perhaps the way for you is to remember yourself as a baby and sense the playfulness and magic that would allow you to go from the floor to standing. Take all the time you need, giving yourself permission to explore the most circuitous path imaginable.

To reenergize yourself after this internal journey, slowly allow yourself to feel the calm vibrations that pulse through your body and sense how the energies in your body connect to the rhythms and pulses of the universe. Slowly begin to allow your arms, shoulders, neck, and head to slightly pulse or jiggle. Then allow your torso to share in the motion, beginning with small movements, and gradually allow the backs of your thighs and calves and your buttocks to wiggle, giggle; release like Jell-O. Remember, no one is looking, so go for what feels good.

Gradually turn your attention to how this experience is like a loop, standing, moving to the floor, and rising again. Allow the cyclic, circular images and associations that may come to you to resonate within your body. We have the ability to move with more ease, grace, and possibility, but we must first attend to our body clues, which we have generally long ago forgotten or learned to ignore. When given time and attention, the effortlessness we once knew within our bodies can easily be rediscovered.

Mindfulness

My state
Angry and stiff
Stiff and angry

It takes a lot of energy to stay
Angry and stiff.

—*Marianne Adams*

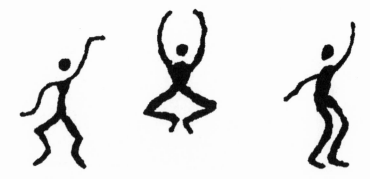

© Rhonda Peterson

Tenderness and Dignity

A tender heart
is not an affliction

dignity comes
to the tendering one

Soften your gaze
at the mirror of imperfection

dissolve those unkind words
in the clear pond of your being

and wrap the soft mantle
of mercy round your shoulders

for the wild thing that you are
needs a blessing

a long drink
from the melon breast of the moon

a saucer of milk
placed at the back door

to let you know
you're not forgotten

Tender yourself
like the kitten you are

the depth of your hunger
is known by none other

than you

—Kirtan Coan

(see plate #3)

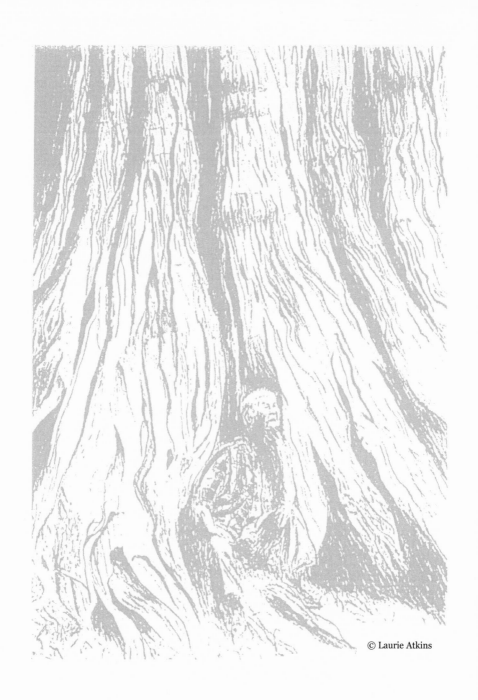

© Laurie Atkins

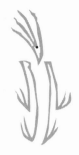

Chapter 5

INSEARCH

*B*eing present within the depths of ourselves can feel both mysterious and familiar. In this place, there is paradox: we are still, and at the same time, we resonate with all the universal motion that surrounds, cradles, and engulfs us. We often feel very connected to the larger world and yet are alone. Both relaxed and focused, we could easily lose track of time or feel as if time and space have been momentarily suspended.

In this stage of the cycle, nonlinear intuition freely guides us; we enter an altered state of consciousness. Sometimes our discoveries come from kinesthesia, spurred on by a body-felt sensation or an emotional realization. Here, knowledge comes to us on many levels, crossing the senses, shapeshifting from visual sensations to forgotten dreams to fragmented rational memories.

In this centered, core state, the learning is often profound and transformational. We are privy to an awareness that is not always apparent in the midst of our ordinary, daily life. In this state, we sometimes feel a sense of deep intuitive wisdom and appreciate a capacity for communion with forces larger than ourselves.

In this chapter, we share poetry, dreams, imagery and music, and body-sensing experiences because the learning that comes in this part of the cycle is often nonverbal, subterranean, and abstruse. With practice, openness, and receptivity, these modalities can access material from the unconscious mind. Often, it is a place where written words can express only partial meanings, where rational thoughts, visceral memories, feelings, and images collide. In this collision and the subsequent reconfigurations, we may feel that we are tasting shadows and touching light.

(see plate #4)

Tasting Shadows, Touching Light

In silence, begin the insearch—
hollow in
    to the place of dreams,
        where floating follows mystery
           wandering gives way to chaos,
              and unexplained shadows are cradled in
              rosewater.

        What resonates, stays,
          long into the night?

    Dreams transform wild, hidden terror—
we fall, spin, stand frozen in the night,
    we fall and spin,
        are carried into dancing.

In the stillness, recognition is borne of essence,
    Re-membering flows from letting go.
Soul knows the way.
    Attending, distancing,
        distractions abound—
Soul brings us back.

    Witness: secrets soaring

    Witness: truth & synchronicity

        Witness: the unknown

    Tasting Shadows
    Touching Light.

        —*Marianne Adams*

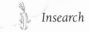

The Magic of Dreams

Facing the challenges of life would be very difficult without the wisdom of dreams.

- Someone involved in a dispute with a friend wakes up singing, "You say Either, I say eIther, let's call the whole thing off" and realizes their intention to end the relationship is petty and misguided.

- A woman trying to make a decision about graduate school has a series of dreams directing her to the right fit for her needs, desires, and abilities.

- A man about to enter into a contract with a particular company awakens from "some sort of dream" knowing only not to sign the contract. Later he finds out that the company is a front for a drug operation.

- A man feeling the burdens of raising a child with a disability has a dream in which he sees that child as a powerful bird upon which he must depend for his own flight.

Experiences leading to better relationships, projects completed, better courses, healthier diets, insights into problem solving, and physical remedies all come from a variety of dreams. Such richness may discourage our ever telling anyone, "Just forget it. It's just a dream." Precognition, important warnings, greater perspective, healing, and transpersonal experiences can and do come through dreams.

According to sleep research, we all dream several times each night. However, only some of us choose to remember our dreams. Can you imagine taking nightly journeys and encountering people, places, and experiences capable of changing who we are in incredibly powerful and wondrous ways, then choosing to forget those experiences because they are "just dreams"? Countless wise people make nightly preparations, laying out their journals, carrying important questions into the infinitely vast world of dreams. They know that in this world the possibilities for understanding and encountering are truly limitless and that these possibilities have the power to bring gifts beyond our grandest expectations.

Courageous dreamers work through conflict by facing and ultimately embracing their nightmares. Later these same dreamers may find themselves more than rewarded for their efforts with awe-inspiring and transpersonal experiences. People tell of waking in tears, feeling unworthy of the gifts they have received in their dreams.

Friends who barely knew each other learn to share parts of themselves that they are only beginning to discover as they tell each other dreams. They leave these encounters with new regard for the friend and a sense of awe at the connections made possible through shared dreams.

We are a dreaming people, and it is through our dreams that we can come to appreciate the depth of being. Write your dreams, share your dreams, draw your dreams, act out your dreams, sculpt your dreams, sing and dance your dreams. Never, ever say, "It was just a dream."

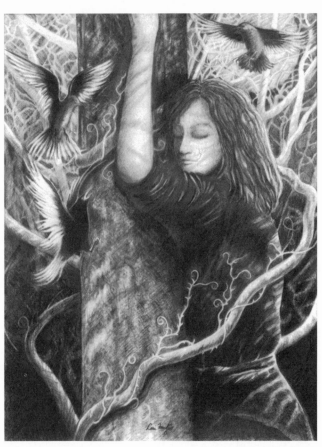

© Lori Fowler-Hill

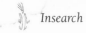

Spirit Guide

This dream began and ended with a unique and beautiful image. It was a cat, whose fur was multi-colored, like a parrot! The only thing this glorious creature did in the dream was stare at me with its intense eyes. There was a feeling that it was penetrating me with its stare. I had an amazing feeling— becoming one with this gorgeous animal.

The mask is my attempt to become one with this sleek, sly, colorful, and curious being in my waking existence.

—Liza Shaw

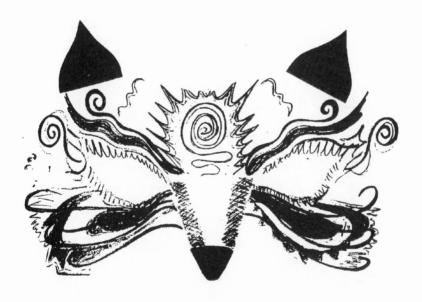

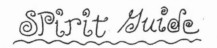

EXPLORATION
Working with Dreams

Dreams are the creation of the imagination, the proof that we are all artists, and there are many creative ways to work with them.

Dai's Approach:

The noted psychotherapist Bingham Dai (1997) emphasizes respect and simplicity in working with dreams. He emphasizes that the function of dreams is to reveal our own deepest wisdom and that although dream symbols may be universal, cultural, and personal, only the dreamer knows the true meaning of the dream. Dai suggests the following steps to work with a dream:

- Tell or write a dream story. Include the date. Write any afterthoughts that come to you.

- Review the events of the day.

- Make free associations to all elements of the dream. What does this make you think of?

- Identify the feeling tone of the dream.

- Make any connections to your current issues or problems in living.

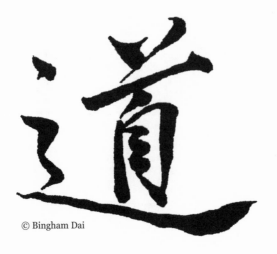

© Bingham Dai

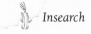

Other Approaches:

TTAQ: Title, Theme, Affect, Question

- Title the dream.
- Write the theme of the dream.
- What is the main thing happening?
- Identify the feeling(s) you, as the dreamer, experienced while dreaming.
- What question is this dream (or this dream symbol) asking of you?

Choose a powerful or mysterious symbol and try one or more of the following:

- Write a cinquain (see chapter 6) using the symbol as the one word of the first line.
- Draw the symbol. With a partner, hold the drawing in front of your face and respond to the following questions in first person:

    Who are you? ("I am a..."). Be specific and concrete.

    What do you feel?

    What do you want?

    What do you feel toward [dreamer's name]?

    What do you want to say to [dreamer's name]?

- Create a dialogue between the symbol and yourself. Take turns assuming the perspective of each and speaking in first person, that is, saying, "I..." from that perspective. For further assistance in creating this dialogue or in moving through conflicts that may emerge, see Faraday's Dream Game (1974).

Take the role of a character or symbol in the dream. Move and speak from this new perspective. Notice how you feel and what you want.

SOLO VOICE
Dream of Transformation

A forty-year-old male therapist's dream: I was aware of a tree stump in a meadow. Next to the stump, walking awkwardly, was an eagle. On a ridge behind the stump was an imposing, but oddly artificial, bull with its back in flames. The eagle jumped up onto the stump and, twirling, became an osprey who took wing. At that moment the back of my own head appeared low in the dream-frame, watching as the osprey flew off toward the mountains. I awoke both agitated and exhilarated.

I woke with the phrase "the stump of Jesse" in my mind. The biblical quote (Isaiah 11: 1, 6, & 9) is:

> *There shall come forth a shoot from the stump*
> *of Jesse, and a branch shall grow out of his roots...*
> *The wolf shall dwell with the lamb, and the leopard*
> *shall lie down with the kid...[and] they*
> *shall not hurt or destroy in all my holy mountain.*

That was exciting because I was recovering from a divorce and was living with a new partner and had begun to write again after a long hiatus. The new shoot seemed like a good sign, new life after the death of a marriage and the presence of a good deal of numbness. As for the eagle, I'm a bird-watcher but at that time had never seen an eagle on the ground. However, the dream image was exactly like what I later saw in Alaska. I felt the eagle on the ground as a taunt, reflecting an accusation that I was the Puer Aeternas, the eternal boy. The association began in thinking about Ganymede carried off to Zeus—not the homosexual element but the fact that Ganymede is eternally a youth serving the adult master. Still, that was old news and not nearly as exciting as the image of the bull with its back in flames nor as disturbing as the fact that the bull was artificial (extremely male, but not real!). I loved the power of the image but again wondered if it amounted to a self put-down, the artificial male, but honestly, that just didn't feel right. When nothing else came to me, I looked up mythic bulls and immediately found Apis and then Ptah, the god of the arts who entered a heifer as celestial fire and was reborn. Hathor, with huge horns, was the great goddess of Egypt who gave birth to the sun. She is sometimes shown as having the sky and the boats of the sun (one led by the morning and one by the evening star) on her belly, presumably because she swallowed the sun at night and gave birth to it in the morning. So the image of the "bull" was both masculine and feminine, and since Ptah was god of the arts, I saw another positive sign. In fact, it almost immediately came to me that Ptah was an anagram for Path, and that perhaps my path was involved with the arts—creative activity.

The osprey and the eagle are similar birds (bald eagle— obvious for me—is a fish-eating raptor, as is the osprey) and that was odd. Also odd was the fact that the osprey twirled in the air like a dancer as the transformation took place. I looked up osprey without luck, but under hawk, I found that boys of Malekula whirl and wave their arms like a hawk when they receive a new name in their initiation ceremony. That struck me (Ptah > Path and I > "artist," my new name). The threefold image of transformation (stump > new growth; eagle > osprey; the bull as an image of or vehicle for rebirth) moved me profoundly. Furthermore, the image of the bird flying toward the mountains suggested a spiritual aspect to the artistic pursuit. I then drew the individual images and the whole picture a number of times until I had a satisfactory representation. I also very soon thereafter completed an opera libretto, wrote a batch of poetry, gave a long reading at a local art gallery, and began again taking lessons on the trumpet and playing in a band—which I did for six more years. In fact, I have in a sense lived out that dream for the past twenty years.

—Jay Wentworth

EXPLORATION
Experiencing Your Creative Space...Music

Find a quiet place free from interruptions or distractions. All you need in this space is quiet, physical comfort, your journal, a CD player, and one of the following recommended CDs. (A stereo with high-quality speakers is nice, but a personal stereo with headphones will also do.) Make yourself physically comfortable with your music equipment prepared and close by.

Take a few moments to settle in. Take care that your body is comfortable. Set aside any worries, lists of "things to do," or other mental chatter that may be cluttering your thoughts. Take a few deep breaths to center yourself and prepare for the experience to come.

Turn your attention to your imagination. In your imagination, see yourself in your own creative space. It may be a space you have been to before or a space given to you by your imagination just for today. It may be indoors or outside. It may be just what you expected or a total surprise. It may come as a place, a color, a feeling, or a body sensation. Simply allow whatever space emerges to be there. Do not try to create it or force it. Do not judge it or attempt to change it. If there is more than one space, simply allow them to move through until one has emerged for you. Honor it for the gift that it is.

As you begin the music, allow the music to be with you in this space as you explore. Allow the music to lead you. If you find that the music takes you into a different space from that in which you began, allow it to do so. Simply be with the music and allow it to lead you as you explore your creative space.

Start the music now.

When the musical selection has ended, turn off the stereo and allow yourself to spend a few moments more in your space bringing your experience to a close. You may want to draw or write in your journal. Allow your images or words to express the essence of your experience. Know that this is your space and that you can return here whenever you want to; it is always here.

Recommended Musical Selections:

Samuel Barber, *Adagio for Strings.* (Baltimore Symphony with Zinman)

Claude Debussy, *Danses sacree et profane.* (New Philharmonic Orchestra with Boulez)

Franz Joseph Haydn, "Adagio" from *Cello Concerto in C.* (Baltimore Symphony with Zinman or St. Louis Symphony with Slatkin)

Ludwig van Beethoven, "Adagio" from *Piano Concerto No. 5.* (Royal Philharmonic with Previn, pianist: Ax)

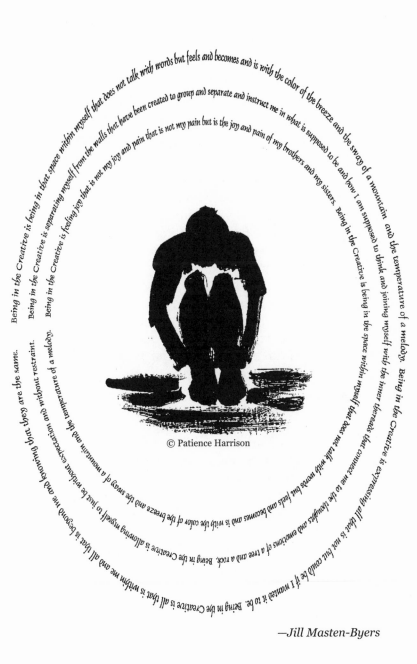

Being in the Creative is being in that space within myself that does not talk with words but feels and becomes and is with the color of the breeze and the sway of a mountain and the temperature of a melody. Being in the Creative is expressing all that is not but could be if I wanted it to be. Being in the Creative is all that is within me and all that is beyond me and knowing that they are the same. Being in the Creative is separating myself from the walls that have been created to group and separate and instruct me in what is supposed to be and how I am supposed to think and joining myself with the inner thereous that connects me to the thoughts and emotions of a tree and a rock. Being in the Creative is allowing myself to just be without explanation and without restraint. Being in the Creative is feeling joy that is not my joy and pain that is not my pain but is the joy and pain of my brothers and my sisters. Being in the Creative is being in the space within myself that does not talk with words but feels and becomes and is with the color of the breeze and the sway of a mountain and the temperature of a melody.

© Patience Harrison

—*Jill Masten-Byers*

Centersearch

Crouching at the edge
of age fortyplus, I am
seeking my womanbones,
womanvoice, womanblood.
I am warming myself
at the bellyfire ignited
millennia ago and stoked
by one woman, then another.
I am mating with the soulcells
of a familiar other, this man
in my lovebed. I am asking
new questions about his manmuse.
I am dancing with the holyghosts
of womenwolvesmendogsdoves
butterfliesbears cavorting
inside me. I am reaching out
to cloudsounds, leaflights,
starpulses, stonelickings:
I am taking it all in, cradling
the fullness, waiting for my
waters to break. Ready, stretching,
opening, opening, opening

—Sharon A. Sharp

Chapter 6

FINDING VOICE

To sing, dance, paint, to speak from the inside out, to let go to the flow that is not about the self but something bigger—this is the creative process for which we have been preparing. It is for this truth-telling that we have made a sacred space. In this space of stillness and safety, trust, and compassion we can find voice to stand to the truth of who we are.

Finding voice, finding a way to express our deepest selves, can be done in many ways, as many ways as there are possibilities for creative acts. I think of friends who find voice in their gardens, in the food they prepare for friends and family, in the handmade cards they send to others, acts made sacred by intention and care. I think of a white-haired Catholic sister I met in Minnesota who grows her own flowers, dries them, and incorporates them into little handmade candles. It is not the form itself that matters, but the depth and integrity of the expression. We are always "moved" in the presence of such expression. (See Plate #5.)

All creative expression begins in the body. In this world we are embodied creatures. In movement and dance the body itself becomes the art form. Everything alive is in motion; everything alive is vibrating. Our bodies are ensembles of rhythm—the breath, the heartbeat, the pulsing of blood through our veins.

In story, in movement, in song we claim the power of the arts to witness the authentic expression of who we are, and we claim the power of that artistic expression for healing. We know the capacity for such expression to move us out of the stuck places, to comfort and heal, and to move us toward wholeness.

In this section we focus on ways of giving voice to the truth of our own experience. We explore the power of word and story to give shape and meaning to the essential questions of our lives: Who are we? What is the meaning of our lives? How are we to live in relationship with each other and with the natural world? All of the teachings of the great philosophies, religions, and cultures of the world are contained in story. What is the story we are living now?

The Imperative of Song

You who have only heard
The sound
Of tension
From your throat,
Know that the ancient ones
Mapped their land by song.
To sing is to get somewhere;
Know that song
Is your incarnation,
Whether an aria
A prayer
Or a single word.

To speak from the inside out
Is to witness
To your own humanity.

Listen,
The heartbeat
Of an ancient beast

Moves through you.
You can only listen
And love it.
And weep,
The sound of your own voice
Singing.

—Sally Atkins

Misknowmer

I have a strong thing to tell
you
But fear you will mis-know
me
As arrogant.
I am soft spoken;
Did I have any say-so
In the shape of my mouth?
I tell you, despite my doubts
That I am worth listening
to.
My soft sounds create
Iron in the words I make.

—Catherine Cope

Poem Drum

This is who I am,
A poem drum
Drumming rhythm,
Drumming deep,
Beating with words,
Beating images of the natural state
Of me, of we
Who beat our lives
One breath at a time.
Heartfelt drum
Of the ancients,
Pulsing connection
Of then and now,
Pulsing connection
Of why and how,
I speak
With your
Resonance.

—Mark Larsen

EXPLORATION
The Power of Naming

To name is: to create meaning
to call into being in the present
    moment
to evoke emotion
to alter consciousness
to shape reality
to stand to the truth of one's own experience

In writing about the archetype of the magician in *The Hero Within* (1989), Carol Pearson says that it is the power of the magician to name. In Native American traditions, Spider Woman, or Thought Woman, names things; and as she names them, they appear. For Native people, words are not symbols for something else. What is named is made manifest and called into the reality of the present moment. This idea suggests the need for reflection and careful attention to what we call into being with our words.

While nonverbal expression is the most authentic, direct, primitive, and universal form of communication, it is in the realm of language that understanding is clarified and meaning is refined. Language shapes our consciousness. Words are magic. They conjure things.

The work of therapy is that of storytelling and story receiving. Telling one's story is a form of naming. It is the privilege of the therapist to bear witness to story. But stories are more than individual. All of the teachings of the world's greatest spiritual and philosophical traditions are contained in story. The stories we are living in our lives are multifaceted. All of the stories we know, the fairytales, the ancient myths and legends, the stories from the Bible and other religious traditions live in us. Stories teach us who we are and how we are to live, in relationship with each other and with the natural world.

The stories of our lives connect seemingly unrelated events, meaningful coincidences, and chance relationships. Carl Jung (1954) named these meaningful coincidences synchronicity. The words on the following page name many concepts that may be themes, lessons, and blessings in life. Close your eyes. Let your finger drift over the page and arrive, by chance, at a word. How does your word fit into the story of your life? What associations do you have with this word? What feelings does it evoke? What

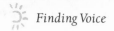

experiences do you connect with it? What symbol expresses this word for you?

abundance   *integrity*   presence   *wonder*   **desire**

magic   beauty   *joy* **acceptance**

memory   belonging   center   sanctuary

commitment   *harmony*   reclaiming

journey   connection   **expression**   synchronicity

consciousness   tenderness   courage

gratitude   unity   **discernment**

breath   spirit   **energy**   source   **flow**

curiosity   **generosity**

delight   **growth**   strength

tranquility   healing   attention

respect   **honor**   inspiration   *wisdom*

intuition   circle   **kindness**

metamorphosis   **humor**   nature

opening   balance   passion   transformation

nurturance   *intensity*   *truth*   reflection

refuge   **grace**   alchemy

serenity   *life-force*   compassion

ground   shelter   solitude

awe   spiral   **freedom**

stillness   *trust*   forgiveness

heart/mind   understanding

possibility   wholeness

benevolence   *intention*   surrender

mystery   renewal

Today's Story

About being mildly discontent
slightly overwhelmed, just somewhat
edgy, never quite sure. This
precarious state is in the undefined
widely encompassing zone of
neurosis with hidden fears
partially on the horizon uncomplicated
by an oh so close state of
almost there. That is, next to
almost right but and of course
always could be a little better.
Although in due time there are
improvements to catch up to
  And certainly the realization
of all that is not now, not then,
ever known or to be understood.

If time could ever frame two
sides at once claiming youth
as it's muse and experience
as another. . . .

If's are always a cornerstone in the everpresent state of malcontent the basis for the onlys formed by the windows of what could have been

The end.

Marianne Adams

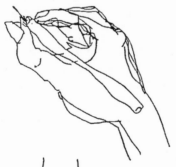

Written & drawn with my now more than ever used but still infrequent Right Hand

EXPLORATION
Today's Story

The idea for this piece arose from a mindfulness exercise in which I was struggling to use my nondominant hand for everyday actions. Research suggests that brain patterning and functioning can by altered by changing your dominant hand while writing (Edwards, 1979). Not only does the practice bring awareness to an often overlooked everyday action, but it also can influence writing style, word choice, receptivity, and perspective.

Write a story with your nondominant hand.

Finding Voice through Limits

Sometimes a glimpse of our own unconscious may yield puzzling or mysterious images. Other times, we may have experiences that are so profound or expansive as to defy our attempts to share them or even acknowledge their reality. During these times we have the opportunity to explore the power of limits, the paradoxical freedom that comes from having restrictions (May, 1975).

Limits contain. They provide boundaries that allow us to grasp the essence of an image or experience and bring that essence into the light of day. They help to frame an experience or a portion of an experience so that we have the opportunity to examine it more closely, to see it from other perspectives, and to claim its gifts more fully.

We may choose limits in any modality. In music, we may limit the sounds to specific scales, modes, keys, notes, or instruments. In movement, we may limit the parameters to include only a specific body part, a confined space, or an arbitrary amount of time. In visual art, we may limit the media, the colors, or the size. In poetry, we may limit syllables, words, lines, or form.

The simple structures of cinquain, haiku, and mandala drawings offer the possibility for such containment. Through the power of limits, it is possible to begin with a single word for the image or experience and move to a deeper understanding, toward acknowledging and claiming the gift.

EXPLORATION
Creating a Cinquain

Choose a word about which you want a deeper understanding or insight. Use that word as the first line and develop the following structure. Use each word no more than once.

Line 1:   One word.

Line 2:   Two words that describe line 1.

Line 3:   Three action words ending in *-ing* that describe line 1. What is it doing?

Line 4:   A four-word phrase or sentence that sums lines 1-3 or further describes line 1.

Line 5:   One word, a metaphoric synonym for line 1.

Example:

> *Purple*
> *Awesome, expansive*
> *Calling, bestowing, uplifting*
> *The way is prepared*
> *Anointed*

EXPLORATION
Creating a Mandala

The mandala is art in the form of a circle. Drawing within the confines of a circle can help us focus on the essence of an experience. Lightly draw a circle a bit smaller than the width of the paper. Using crayons or oil pastels, draw within the circle the feeling of a dream or experience. It is not necessary to draw concrete images; simply allow the feeling to manifest itself in color or form. (see also plate #1)

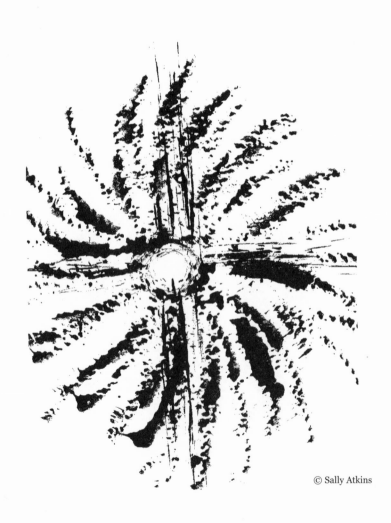

© Sally Atkins

EXPLORATION
Creating a Haiku with Traditional Structure

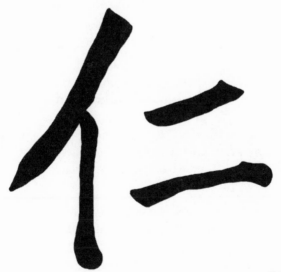

Choose a symbol or image about which you desire clarity. It may be a dream image, a word, a feeling, or any other experience. Using the following structure, explore the essence of the symbol:

Line 1:   5 syllables
Line 2:   7 syllables
Line 3:   5 syllables

Example:

> *Dark murky water*
> *Settles into clarity*
> *Shining gold revealed.*

> *Shining gold nugget*
> *Calling from dark recesses*
> *Offering its light.*

EXPLORATION
Creating a Haiku with Nontraditional Structure

Instead of following the 5/7/5 form, you can write haiku by focusing on spontaneity and on keen observations in nature. Go outside or look out your window, and then write several short sentences about what you see. Here are some examples:

> *A triangle of snow remains in the boulder's shadow.*
> *Purple blackberry stems wave in the wind.*
> *The creek runs over mossy rocks.*
> *The stump has become an ant condo.*
> *Amidst tight rhododendron buds, one is splitting.*
> *A roughed grouse feather spins in the laurel.*

Now form a new image by linking any of the two sentences with the word while or as. For instance:

> *A triangle of snow remains in the boulder's shadow while*
> *A roughed grouse feather spins in the laurel.*

This combination emphasizes stillness and movement, as well as hanging on and letting go. Another possibility would be:

> *The stump has become an ant condo while*
> *Amidst tight rhododendron buds, one is splitting.*

The second combination emphasizes the press of life, the power of creation in the face of death or other obstacles.

Next, consider a dream you have had, an image you have drawn, or a movement exercise you have done and write several observations about it. Then join two observations by using while or as, and change some of the wording if that would make the comparison or link clearer. For example, in response to two mandalas a man had drawn (one with the dominant right hand on white paper and the other with the left on black paper), he wrote the following observations:

> *One goes outside in and the other goes inside out.*
> *The dark one is more fluid, the light more rigid.*
> *There are more colors in one, but the other is more intense.*
> *Doors and directions; a winding path.*

He then connected two observations and described his thoughts.

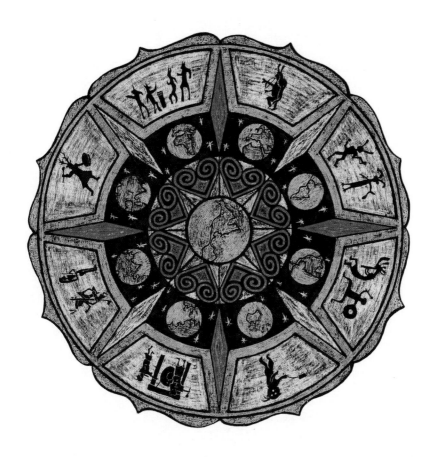

Plate #1. Untitled. ©Lindley C. Sharp

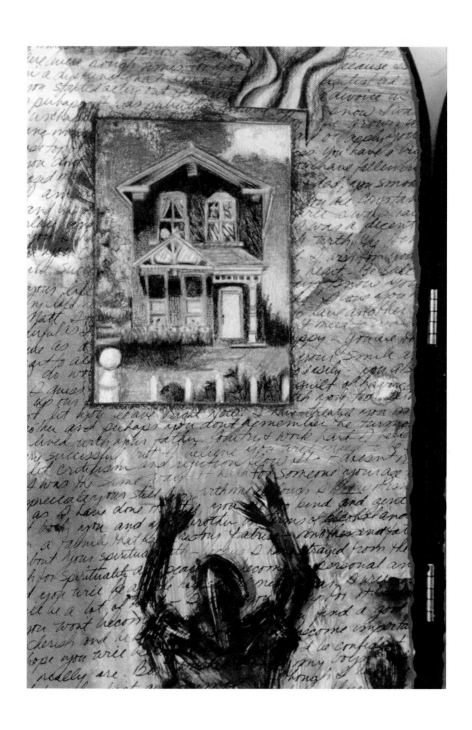

Plate #2. *Home on Fire.* ©Lori Fowler-Hill

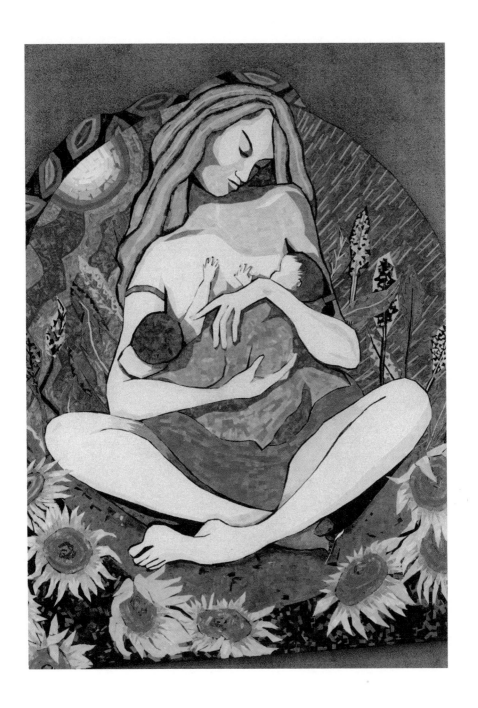

Plate #3. *Demeter*. ©Lori Fowler-Hill

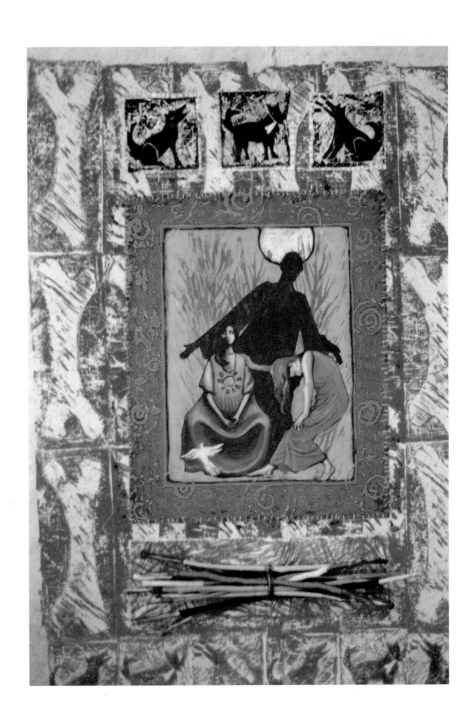

Plate #4. *Together Not Broken.* ©Lori Fowler-Hill

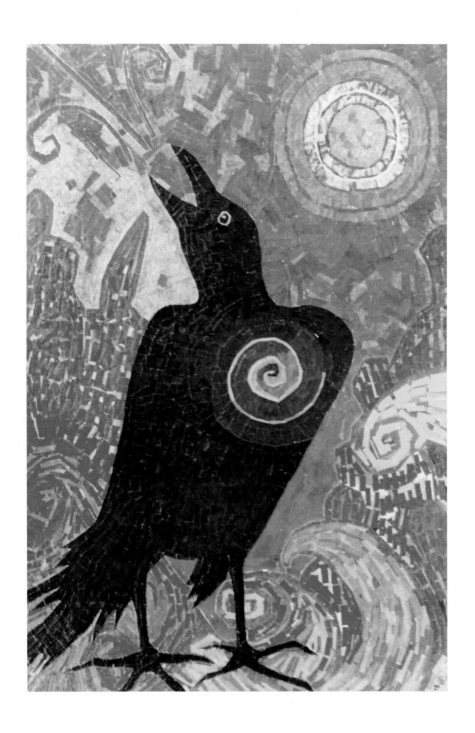

Plate #5. *Get Back, no. 1.* ©Lori Fowler-Hill

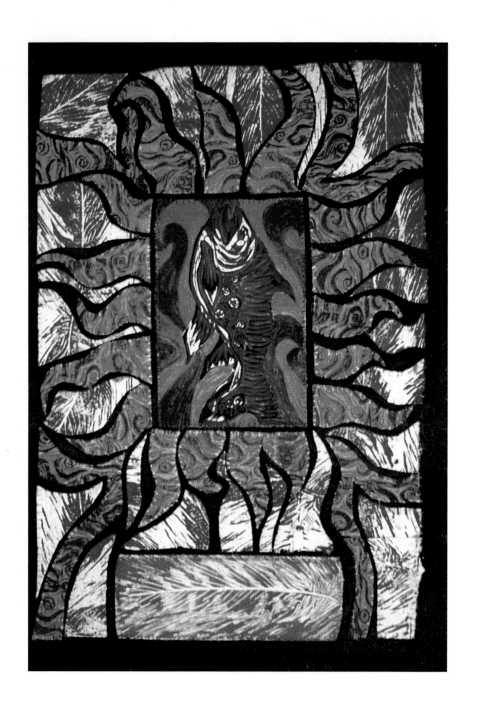

Plate #6. *Union.* ©Lori Fowler-Hill

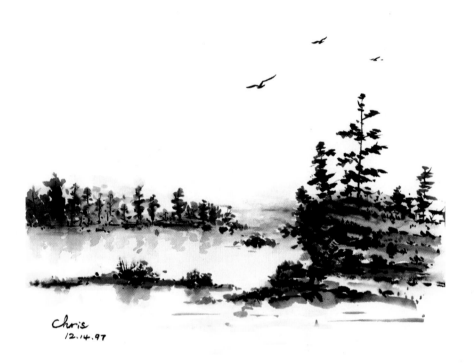

Plate #7. Untitled. ©Wang Yanbin

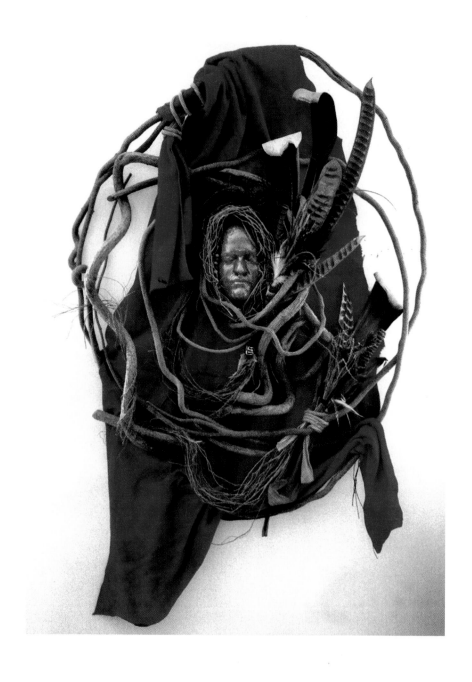

Plate #8. *Spirit Shield*. ©Toni Carlton

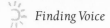

First response:

> Fluid dark is more intense; light more full of color.

> It was nice to take ownership of aspects of each mandala that I liked rather than feel the initial disgust with the first one.

Second response:

> Going in is harder for me; coming out more secure—lost without center, hard to let go.

> I realized that my mind (rational training and expectations) is divorced from my emotional and artistic center to an extent I had not previously known. This leads me to consider (try out ways of) integrating them more.

By playing with ways of connecting your statements, you often can uncover or even stumble into new insights about the original experience, as well as your current thoughts, feelings, and actions.

Third response:

> I prefer the winding, more mysterious path to the usual set of doorways and directions, yet my life is more controlled by the latter. I'm excited by the implied invitation to change.

Chant

The Muslim calls to prayer. The Christian monk chants his way through the Mass. The field worker brings rhythm and tone into the muscle fibers of the body so he might more easily accomplish his work. The schoolchild alters her perception of time on a long bus trip with the repetitious "Ninety-Nine Bottles of Beer." The contemporary Christian worshipper cycles through countless "Alleluias." The highly skilled Tibetan Buddhist produces very low tones and corresponding overtones in harmonic drones altering his environment for devotion. The Hindu raises his voice in ecstatic praise. Our cultures are filled with chant. Chant for worship, chant for work, chant for passing time, chant for the joy of bathing ourselves in vibration. Chant can be a way of informing ourselves about the present condition of our interior being, and it can be a way of altering that condition.

When one begins to chant, she may find a quiver in her voice. As she connects with the breath, this quiver may even out into a steady tone. Her entire being settles as connection with the breath allows her to accomplish her tonal intent—no small lesson. Particular affirmations may be embodied vocally, giving the cells of the body informed vibratory consent to move in a particular direction.

It is said that "when one sings, he prays twice." The power of the voice as a tool for uniting the human will is evident not only in the voice of the military commander but more subtly and perhaps even more powerfully in chant. By chanting, one seizes the opportunity to align the physical, mental, emotional, and spiritual selves for a common good.

EXPLORATION
Chanting Discoveries

Find a space where you will feel free to use your voice however you please. Sit in a comfortable position with the spine erect. Close your eyes and begin to listen. Is there a predominant tone to be heard within? Can you find a syllable or vowel by which to join with that tone, or is there a more significant experience in just listening internally? As you intone your particular sound or as you listen internally, are there images or physical sensations that accompany your tone? Does your body want to sway or move forward and back? Where do you find the tone connecting most strongly to your body? Are there other tones that want to come with your sound? Do you find yourself wanting to sing small phrases? Do the phrases have words? Do they take form in ways that are expected or somewhat surprising? Do you want to accompany this musical movement with walking or dance? Stay with your vibratory creation as long as you like. Let it evolve and resolve however it may. When it seems appropriate, allow your experience to come into silence. Stay with this silence as long as you wish.

When you are ready, begin to reconnect to your external environment. What are the sounds in your environment? Are there birds chirping? Can you hear traffic or a refrigerator or a distant door slam? What do you hear? How are you different from when you entered the experience? What do you know that you did not know before the chant? Having had the experience, what might you wish to do, write, draw, give, or create?

SOLO VOICE
Dreaming the Gift of a Song

You are the sea, the deep, the blue to me
You are the mist and stars above
You are the water and the mystery
You'll be my true and only love.

Sometimes the very process of expression, of giving voice, results in healing. At one very painful, low point in my life, I was given a song in a dream that became the turning point in my healing cycle.

I was grieving the loss of a relationship that had been very short but very intense. During the grieving process, I had been journaling and painting, giving expression to lots of feelings. On the evening before the dream came, I had written a long letter to the man I had been involved with, hoping for some sense of closure. I planned to hold the letter for a few days and then, if it still felt appropriate, to send the letter.

Very early the next morning, I awoke from a dream suddenly. As I was lying in bed thinking about the dream, I gradually became aware of some music in the background of the dream. I began to hum the melody as I lay in bed. Soon I realized that it was a melody I didn't recognize. I sat up and lit a candle next to the bed and tried to write the melody into my journal. (This was difficult, as I don't write in musical notation.)

As I put the melody into the journal, I began to hear words for the song. I began to write the words as they came in couplets and verses and phrases. I just wrote it all down as fast as I could.

> *I love the tides that brought you close to me*
> *I blessed the dawning of that day*
> *I grieve the loss of all you've been to me*
> *I feel it flowing all away.*
>
> *I tried to hold your water close to me*
> *And of your love I ne'er did tire*
> *But your wet ways have been the death of me*
> *These bitter tears have drowned my fire.*

A couple of hours later, I went to a piano to pick out chords. Then I began to work with the lyrics, arranging the couplets and verses into some kind of order. By late afternoon, I had the whole song—the melody, the chords, the lyrics.

Writing the song was extremely healing. The process of giving voice to my feelings allowed me to fully own my experience and to find some sense of compassion for my situation. The song had room to contain my unique pain and the universal experience of lost love. The song helped me see the bigger picture and fully experience my own situation.

I remember the making of that song as the beginning of movement out of grief and toward healing. I did not send the letter for closure. The song became personal closure for me. Sometime later I sang the song for friends who had known of the relationship. At that point I felt the healing was complete.

> *Now I'm the sea, the blue the mystery*
> *I am the old, I am the new*
> *Where there is water, love...remember me*
> *And know my love for you was true.*

—*Terri Chester*

Freehand

When you go searching
for songs, open
your hands. Let
the widening circles
of time hum in your
palms and ripple outward.
Feel the patterned tunes
seeping through earth,
tumbling from clouds.
Add your own. Celebrate
the unending revolutions
of sounds shared.

—Sharon A. Sharp

SOLO VOICE
Finding Voice, Making Dance

To be a choreographer, you must reserve judgment—like in the movies, it requires a willing suspension of disbelief.

Engage in the process
  One step at a time
There are many choices
An infinite number of ways to go
The most important lesson is to make conscious choices
To know why you chose what you chose

To explore fully your possibilities
In a way that speaks uniquely of your experience,
perspective—
Be ferocious in adding
Your imprint on the world.

For me, there is a kind of uneasy faith that guides the continuation of the process. In the middle, choreography always feels like it becomes a process of uncovering fear. Fear and self-doubt often lead me into a place of darkness that I never quite anticipate going. It is certainly not all about angst, but it is always about growth, and that often comes in awkward, unpredictable ways. It often feels chaotic to go through those times when nothing seems to come or when what I try doesn't quite work.

However, I have found some freedom in facing myself or a group of dancers and saying, "I don't quite know where to go here." It often feels that an out-loud admission releases a block, that I am somehow able to begin again, engage in sensation and be absorbed in the process after making that statement. It is a moment of letting go of past pictures, expectations, and illusions of grandeur. It is also a moment that reminds me...I make dances with a community larger than myself and that working collectively with a group of dancers lends more creative support than I could ever tap individually—if I just have the courage and trust to ask for collective vision. Then mystically, the creative process creeps on ...by trial and error, by process of elimination, by whimsy and pain, by leading me where I most need to go...serendipity.

I have found it works best if I allow myself to be guided and informed by the process and unattached to the outcome. And, since dancers tend to be an impatient lot, I find I need to encourage them at this point not to lose faith or be disconcerted by all the variations and discards we have gathered. The renditions, in bits and pieces, form the pentimento of the piece. The peeled layers will add a richness and depth to the piece that can be felt, if not always seen. The pulling together of the piece ultimately comes from the dancers' experience, their investment in the process, and the community we make while dancing together.

—Marianne Adams

Dance is the expression of the human condition.
You are saying this is who I am. It is not about adding on,
doing more and more. It is about letting go of everything that
is not essential and then saying...this is still who I am.

—Abby Fiat

EXPLORATION
Owning the Gift

Perhaps the only way to find your own creative voice is to watch for it, listen for it, and allow it to find you. The following experience is designed to be done after "Experiencing Your Creative Space...Music" (see chapter 5); however, that is not an absolute prerequisite. If you have a sense of your space, you may want to proceed with the following experience.

Find a quiet place free from interruptions or distractions. All you need in this space is quiet, physical comfort, your journal, a CD player, and one of the following recommended CDs. (A stereo with high-quality speakers is nice, but a personal stereo with headphones will also do.) Make yourself physically comfortable with your music equipment prepared and close by.

Take a few moments to settle in. Take care that your body is comfortable. Set aside any worries, lists of "things to do," or other mental chatter that may be cluttering your thoughts. Also set aside any predetermined expectations of the outcome of this experience. Take a few deep breaths to center yourself and prepare for the experience to come.

Turn your attention to your imagination. In your imagination, see yourself in your own creative space. Notice what there is around you here. There may be objects, colors, feelings, or sounds. Take in all that is here for you.

When the music begins, allow it to be with you in your space and to bring you something—a feeling or a sensation, a color or an object, a word or a phrase, an impulse to do something. Whatever the music brings, honor it without censure or judgment. Simply be with the gift of the music in whatever way seems right for you. When the musical selection has ended, turn off the stereo and allow yourself to spend a few moments bringing your experience to a close. Start the music now.

After the music has ended, you may want to draw or write in your journal. Allow your images or words to express the essence of your experience. For now, simply let the experience be without analysis or interpretation. Savor the gift.

Recommended Musical Selections:

J. S. Bach, "Sinfonia" from *Christmas Oratorio.* (on Music for Relaxation 2: The Romantic Bach, London 440-082-2)

Gabriel Faure, "In Paradisum" from *Requiem.* (Montreal Symphony and Chorus with Dutoit)

Gustav Holst, "Venus" from *The Planets.* (Montreal Symphony with Dutoit)

Maurice Ravel, *Introduction and Allegro.* (Melos Ensemble on London label or Ensemble Wien-Berlin on DDG)

What is a poem?

The admission that I still
Hunger for what disappears
Between the lines,
The ghost of dreams
And banished children,
Although I know that words
Are smaller than images,
This is my blood
Black on this page.
I tell you this:
I will be the interpreter
Of my own experience.
I know now
That nothing in my body lies.

—*Sally Atkins*

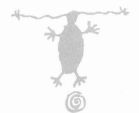

Chapter 7

BRINGING ART INTO LIFE

All the arts that we practice are apprenticeship.
The big art is our life.
—*M. C. Richards*

We literally create ourselves by what we practice: we wire our brains, strengthen muscles, build bone. If we are alive, we are integrated in some ways—not all links may be optimal, but they allow us at least to survive, and that is why, even when we feel terrible, it may be difficult to change. Our bodies and our lives reflect our practices, and our psychospiritual practices, like body lesions, can warp our lives. Still, because they represent the only integration we have, they can also impede new attitudes and behaviors. Fear blocks new integration because it is the primal response to the threat of disintegration, so even the creative integration we expect to foster is a risk, and that risk must be honored into practice. Risk taking (not recklessness) is the ignition for all art and creativity. Moving into the world, into daily life where our habits were formed in the first place seems to risk every new impulse, every new skill and integration. Yet it must be done, so how do we do it chin high, with energy in spite of fear?

In some ways, the gentle technique of becoming aware of breathing may stand for all the work of expressive arts therapy. If we practice awareness of breathing, we feel the in-drawing of air (inspiration), hold and feel the tension build (risk/work), and then experience the pleasure of release (expression). Holding the emptiness (accepting the disintegrated, uninspired state in trust) is the key because that is what allows tension to build (risk/work) until we feel the pleasure of the next inhalation (inspiration). The breathing-in provides the energy and thus the opportunity for integration; the release gives the reward for risking the next round of tension-building work, which is a letting go of the need to immediately refill. But when the refilling comes, we are renewed and rewarded again.

When we are afraid, we hold our breath, so we tend to associate held breath with fear. Thus, practice with held breath works to overcome fear. If we breathe into our fear, we are inspired! By following the simple cycle of breath, we integrate and inspire ourselves; we become creators in order to share our fullness with others, and we become able to experience disintegration, knowing it is the foundation for all creative living (integration).

As we move into living as artists in the world, we can make the cycle of breath our guide and teacher. Developing habits of art such as listening to music we love, making space to throw pots (ha!— yes, that too), drawing, practicing an instrument, cooking for the creativity rather than utility of it, or just being aware of "both/and" as an alternative to "either/or" can aid the inspiration we need to continue the integrative journey toward wholeness. Habits of the arts! They support our lifelong growth.

We may also remind ourselves that moving out is moving in— to community. We may find ourselves speaking up in a PTA meeting or offering to head a committee or starting a club or...who knows—if we knew, it wouldn't be creative. The joy of creative living spills out in the most unexpected ways; the sense of wholeness expands, and risk becomes more and more desirable. Fear is lived into and rewards increase. Wonderfully, others tend to mirror our way of presenting ourselves, so we often experience support for this creative way of living. The continuing process is the integration of fear with joy, self with others. Imagine that!

© Ty Atkins

Just Drink

To hear this poem
do not look at me

Close your eyes
I cannot be seen

I've gone to Calcutta
for monsoon season

loosed my wits to ride
roan ponies in stampede

that the sheer act of living
break the mind of reason

bring me to my knees at the edge
where words wash ashore

Take off your clothes
and run into the sea

You'll taste this poem
in the salt air

see it floating in a green bottle
bound for your lips

Uncork the brew
and drink

don't analyze the recipe
just drink

—Kirtan Coan

EXPLORATION
Projective Autobiography

Put on a piece of music you think you will enjoy for your whole life. Imagine yourself twenty-five years from now. Consider what the world is like—probably not just an extension of the present. Look back over your life and write an autobiography of creative processes in your life. Consider the role of creativity in your personal growth (including spiritual and artistic development), relationships, profession, community life, connection with nature, and so on. Give yourself as many pages as you wish; explore your life; consider regrets, opportunities taken and missed, the development of your vision and abilities. What daily practices have persisted? What relationships have been important to you? What were some of your most creative ideas, projects, relationships, experiences?

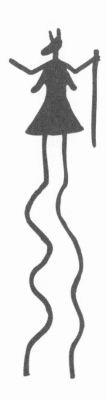

Prayer for Angels

Another early morning awakening
Peace and stillness before the realization
Then the familiar daily free-fall,
That sick,
> *ass over tea-kettle,*
>> *oh-my-god,*
>>> *down-hill drop.*
Stomach and heart changing places.
Anticipation of a bone-shattering crash landing.
Hope for some unpredictable act of grace or
heroism
Some last minute save.
Clutching fear and desperate prayer for angels.
Prayer for wings—mine or theirs—
To float me down gently
Or lift me back up.
Another close call.
Another day to survive
Or to live
Another chance to contemplate
The strange forms that angels may take.

—Terri Chester

SOLO VOICE
Attention and Intention

We are each born with an artist's heart and soul. As children, we all have the ability to experience and appreciate the beauty around us. And in childhood, our ability to live creatively comes more naturally. As we become older and more educated, the ability to create—to be the source of beauty and art—becomes more difficult.

My personal creative process contains a paradox. The creative process requires both the discipline to create a stable container and the flexibility to be able to flow within that container. I need the safety and structure within which to have the freedom to fully express more of who I am and what moves me. Two words come to mind: attention and intention.

Intention involves those elements that create the container: doing our own work, valuing ourselves, creating space and time for the creative process, and practicing a discipline that guides focus and sharpens skills for increasing awareness. Consistent practice of some form of expression is necessary so that when the moment comes to say something, I have the vehicle with which to do it.

And then there is attention. Within the safe container of my intention, I must know how to pay attention to the details of my life: the light on the bedroom wall, the sound of water on rocks, the tightness in my lower back, the color and texture of the cover on my bed, the sensation in my body of wanting to crouch or run or be very still. I must pay attention to what makes me laugh or cry, to what brings me joy or grief or comfort. There must be room for both: intention and attention.

In my experience, it is easier to live a life full of intention. That path is more visible and active, can be seen more easily, and feels good because it involves "doing." Attention is harder because it involves being. It is more passive and less visible, and it can appear unproductive, lazy, and a waste of time. And yet unless I pay attention to what I value, to what moves me, to what wants and needs to be expressed in me, my intention dissipates in a frantic flurry of busyness and unfocused activity.

When I live with more balance, there is a constant tension between the two—between the being and the doing, the intention and the attention. Even as I fully immerse myself in one, I am aware of the constant pull of the other. For me, finding the artistic balance does not necessarily involve finding a static position between the two forces. True balance is about letting the two forces be fully experienced. I have to allow this tension to pull me back toward center if I stray too far in either direction. My process is about valuing each force equally, if differently, and letting each support the other.

—Terri Chester

On a Hillside, the Dragon's Breath

The baseball season has rotted
like this chestnut stump, but hickory
hulls are green; a few orange-breasted
late-packers hieroglyph the air while
homebodied wrens, juncoes and cardinals
stake their claims content to uncover
opportunity in a bear market.

The uphill hike has lit a sugar-maple glow
in legs that threaten to ignite; I catch
in my nose the first burn of winter.

A squirrel runs leaping m's beneath
the casual green of rhododendron
hiding secrets under the secrets
in asparagus-tipped buds. Downed
leaves chatter like old ladies
about their several ills; titmice
give sound to the act of mica
shattering light. An oak limb hangs
snapped loud in the ear of memory,
a relic of the cruel beauty of ice,
and a spider works death-magic in the wind.

I will pause more often.

—Jay Wentworth

SOLO VOICE
Gardening as Daily Practice

Tending a garden as a daily practice is very rich metaphorically and literally. It immediately brings to mind the image of one who cultivates instead of controls. Nature does not allow me to control it, but it teaches me how to work with it in cultivating a productive space. I cannot control what happens in my life, but I can work with each event creatively to view it as a gift from which valuable life lessons are gleaned.

Tending a garden can be difficult, particularly at the beginning, just as a new daily practice can be challenging. Saint Teresa of Avila (1566/1980) exquisitely compares watering a garden to levels of prayer/meditation. She says that when one begins to meditate, doing so is as difficult as physically carrying buckets of water to a dry garden. Later, she says, at a deeper level, one builds aqueducts that allow water to be delivered to the garden continuously. This second level of meditation is deeper, but still laborious. Finally, the rain gently falls on the garden when it is dry, and no human intervention is necessary. This is the third and deepest level of meditation, where a natural rhythm is created and a deep interconnection is established between the inner and the outer self. Cultivating a garden, as in cultivating life, offers a deep and lasting connection with nature's harmonious rhythms.

I find that if I skip my daily practice over a period of three or four days, I have to ask the insightful question, "What is my addiction that is keeping me away from my soul work?" The external world prefers for us not to take this time daily and presents us with many distracting options—work, family, play, general business of life...the list is infinite. I am continually grateful to this process of daily practice/distractions as a way of discovering and deepening my personal growth.

—*Liz Rose*

Touchstones in Our Lives

As we return to our ordinary, everyday lives, our deep experiences in arts and the profound lessons they offer can easily begin to feel surreal. Many of us were taught to minimize frightening imaginal experiences with phrases such as "It was only a dream" or "It was just my imagination." In the days and weeks following the transformative arts experience, we may feel that the experience is less real, less present. This is particularly true following expansive states or experiences of universal consciousness.

To retain the immediacy and potency of the experience, it is often useful to find a way to bring with us a concrete representation of the experience as we move back into our everyday lives. These "touchstones" evoke the recollection of the gestalt of the experience—the feelings, images, words, somatic sensations—and remind us of the reality of where we have been. The touchstone can take any form that will serve this purpose for us. It may be a piece of jewelry that suggests an image, a stone or other object of nature, or the visual art product that emerged from the experience. Sometimes synchronicity will lead us to the work of another artist that captures and evokes recall of our own experience.

Other deep experiences impel us toward daily application in our lives. We may be called to take more time for ourselves, to notice beauty, to be with our children, to value friendships. In these cases, we may choose to act with intention, to consciously apply in our outer lives the learnings from our inner lives. These choices bring wholeness.

Recognition
At curbsides, on roadways,
in postal lines, corridors,
terminals, grocery store aisles
we see them: strangers
with our own longing looks,
our own unspoken hopes, our
own bottomless needs, boundless
capacity for giving. If we,
they do not look away too fast,
the flicker of shared knowing
may glow, sheltered from gusts.

—Sharon A. Sharp

Connecting In, Taking Out

A young woman returns home after a powerful week of music and dance wondering, "How can I stay connected to the way that I am now?" That night she has a dream reminding her to breathe and to stay consciously connected with the breath. This admonition helps her keep a greater sense of life in her daily activities and helps her carry some of the energy of the workshop into her life.

A small child faces frightening dental procedures. As she sits in the dentist's chair and begins to hear the noises of the dental equipment, she remembers to connect with her breath. As her breath deepens, she begins to relax and feel some sense of calm and mastery over her anxiety.

A choreographer who finds herself in the midst of a particularly complex and frustrating challenge provided by tired dancers, inadequate stage space, and a rapidly nearing production deadline begins to hear a line from a poem she had recently written saying, "not by my effort." Almost magically she begins to see the tight space as an opportunity for some close body work. Time seems to expand when she allows the work to claim some much-needed simplicity. The dancers' energy is renewed as they are invited into greater participation in creating the dance. And the final result is a wonderful work that flourishes partly due to the power brought forth by its limitations.

In art, one becomes familiar with the workings of life energy itself. Most golfers know that a golf club cannot be pushed as fast as it will go. Direction is provided in initiating the swing, but the real work is accomplished by much more powerful forces such as gravity and momentum. Often the best work is accomplished by "having the wisdom to get out of the way" (E. Auxier, personal communication, 1997).

Woman on a Rack

Woman on a rack, stretched to her limit,
Gremlin gnawing at her middle.
Acorn mysterious, dark and sealed, waiting, dormant.

"Dear woman," I ask,
"What can I give you?
What do you need?"

"I need to unwind,
To soak up the sun and music.
I need release from the bonds that bind me to this rack."

Release is so scary.
Everything may fall apart.

—Cathy McKinney

A Story

A man
Trying too hard
Holding, hurting, grasping, forcing
Found himself enfolded
By a strong wind
Which forced him to bend.

This bending
Sprang him open,
Throwing life from him
Into All Else That Was.

All Else That Was
Laughed
At what the man offered
Until touched by it.

Then All Else That Was cried
Because it had been joined
By itself and knew itself
To be whole again.

—Harold McKinney

EXPLORATION
I Woman; I Man; I Human

Using any medium (dance, clay, paint, poetry, music, or others), create a piece about what you truly are as your physical gender (try using your nondominant hand and/or a medium with which you are less familiar); then do the same for the opposite gender in you (do this while cross-dressed if you wish and/or work with your dominant hand and/or in a medium with which you are very familiar); then do the same for yourself as human in any fashion that feels right. Media may change or stay the same. When you're done, find the integrative elements (commonalities, complements, contradictions, images, and so on) and share them. This exercise may be done quickly or over time; it may be done alone, in pairs, or with a group. What fears does this work create? What fears does this work alleviate? How does what you discover help you move more confidently into the world? What would you like to do next?

SOLO VOICE
By the Light of the Full Moon

A beautiful image for me growing up on the coast of North Carolina was that of the loggerhead sea turtle who would lay her eggs in a carefully prepared nest on the beach. Then, magically, the babies would hatch on the full-moon nights in June, July, or August, using the light of the moon to guide them to their new home, the sea. I can remember lying in bed on those evenings and feeling a sense of awe and reverence for the baby turtles as they struggled to reach the ocean. The loggerhead's natural cycle of birth continues to nourish me as an adult, even though I am far removed from it geographically. The metaphor of birth and moving toward the light captures the essence of taking art into life for me.

I was deeply thrust into my inner world by a traumatic diagnosis and resulting surgery, which I now reflect upon as the moment of grace in my life. Although my inner journey was painful and difficult, I have only now realized how easy it is to get comfortable deep inside and how much the real challenge lies in taking new energy back into the external world. The point when I realized I had to move back out into life was initiated by a dream of a beautiful sea turtle who had hands and a voice. I painted her, talked with her, and wrote about her. By using the arts, I was able to relate to her healing energy at a deeper level during this critical transitional time. In her own way, she was calling me back out toward the light.

In attempting to be "outward bound," I realized that I was just as vulnerable as a baby sea turtle moving from its nest to the sea. The harsh reality is that many baby turtles don't make it to the ocean on those magical full-moon nights. Their journey is interrupted by predators—crabs, fish, and birds. My new "shell" felt soft, and just as a baby turtle knows that she is facing the most dangerous part of her journey in heading towards the light of the moon, I too was acutely aware of my own existing predators that could easily extinguish the tiny but powerful flame of light that now existed inside of me. Would friends and family accept the new me? Would I be able to make it professionally when I spoke my truth?

I have since learned that people don't like me as much when I stop playing the game of projection and that most people prefer not to hear personal truths spoken. I have learned that I must develop a deep spiritual foundation in order to listen and respond to my own voice and therefore live more fully. Just as the baby turtle trusts her natural instinct to move toward the light of the moon, I too must learn to trust my feminine instinct and intuition to serve as my guide in facing the new challenges that life will inevitably present.

As time progresses, I hope that my shell will harden gracefully. Like the turtle, I have come through a difficult part of the journey—back into the ocean of life. Now it is time to learn how to swim.

(see plate #6)

—Liz Rose

SOLO VOICE
Becoming the Artist Crone

In my professional journey, I am beginning to feel like a grandmother now. After thirty years of psychotherapy practice and twenty-four years of university teaching, I am watching with deep satisfaction as my students become artists, teachers, and clinicians, taking their places in the professional world.

Personally, I am becoming the crone. I find myself less and less interested in the busyness of professional accomplishment and family caretaking that have absorbed these years and more and more drawn to solitude, personal space, time for self-reflection, and a way of life that feels deeply authentic. Day to day, I am seeking a way to live openly, gratefully, a u t h e n t i c a l l y , respectfully, and mindfully.

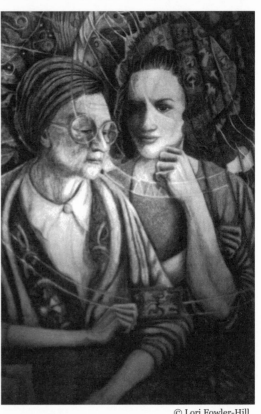

© Lori Fowler-Hill

Now I find that in every class I teach, in every project I undertake, I am reclaiming the reality that I am an artist, deeply engaged in a mysterious process of creativity—moment by moment— participating in a creative process that is much larger than my little self. I am moving toward the place where I can speak and write and live from my heart as well as my head.

—Sally Atkins

It Helps to Remember

Real teaching is about
    Being articulate
    Concise
    Judicious
    Ever So Gentle
    Persistent
        Egoless

Real teaching calls for
    Sharing Wisdom
        Generously
    With Humor
Listening more than we speak
And saying out loud I don't know

Real teaching invites
        Imaginings of the unknowable
        Perspectives of context to emerge

Real teaching demands
    Complete faith . . .

That at least one
    out of every class
        will "really" get it—

It helps to remember
    I was not always the one.

—Marianne Adams

SOLO VOICE
Rituals of Grieving

As a part of our Summer Institute for Expressive Arts in Counseling, held annually at Appalachian State University, I took part in a visual art workshop led by the noted artist and teacher Noyes Capehart Long. At the workshop we drew and painted with found objects—branches, leaves, stones, and flowers. Freed from the need to "draw something in a traditional way," I entered the process deeply. This image, created of black tempera with a pine cone, a feather, and a piece of bark, emerged. I titled it "Grieving." Later, I did not recall the title until a colleague reminded me.

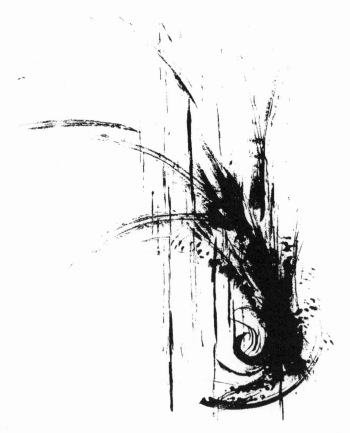

© Sally Atkins

The work of grieving takes time. In our fast-paced lives it is so easy to move on too quickly, reassuming the tasks of ordinary life, sometimes leaving grief work to emerge, unbidden, much later. My mother died nine months before the image "Grieving" emerged. My grieving her loss was not lessened by the fact that her death was not untimely, sudden, or unexpected. The loss of a mother, no matter what the circumstances, is profound. As it was for my mother, letting go is hard for me.

At her funeral six close women friends stood and read a poem that celebrated the strength and mystery of her life. Another close friend played the organ, and we sang her favorite hymns. In a eulogy, I named, as best I could, the truth of who she was for me. My son read the poem that had come to me much earlier, as I anticipated her death.

Leaving

All day I have been memorizing you
As we moved in and out of silence.
All day I have been memorizing you
As you moved in and out of my heart.
I have held the shapes of your words on my tongue,
Tasted slowly, until they slipped away.
What remains is memory.
What remains is memory and love.

I made her casket pall from her antique lace tablecloth and the fragments of an old quilt that she and her mother and sisters had made from feed sacks and cotton from the fields of their farm. I celebrated the combination of her heritage of strength from her Southern Appalachian farm family and her elegance, especially as a teacher. I owned those qualities of strength and elegance I share with her, as well as our not always pretty characteristics of determination and ferocity.

Later I took fragments of lace and quilt to make thank-you cards for the many gifts of love and support I received during that time. I cut and tore the fabrics apart and let the threads unravel at the edges. All of this work was deeply satisfying and healing.

© Sally Atkins

In the months that followed, I continued my grief work with music and imagery and dreamwork. Now, nine months after her death, I realize just how much all of these experiences of poetry, music, ritual making, writing, craft, and painting have held me to honor my mother and my own personal process of grieving. In "Grieving" I see and feel my movement in this process. I own my own growth, opening, and letting go. The process, from the writing of "Leaving" until now, has been almost three years. This writing, too, is part of the process.

—*Sally Atkins*

Heart's Intention

Here is what I want: pure pleasure in prayer,
even as pain continues to shape my soul.

I want to sip the day like morning tea,
to run barefoot through the fields

wearing rain as a silk garment,
at night to bathe in a shower of stars.

I want to live with passion,
to pour out my life as if time

were prolific as summer weeds,
to be extravagant in my giving.

I want to discern the slightest offence
and forgive it right away,

to practice the custody of the lips,
each word carefully chosen.

I want, when death comes,
to know my life was spent

tending the chambers of the wounded heart.

—*Pam Noble*

Body Prayer as Remembering

Breath of Joy
Remembering that the breath is our literal connection with what seems beyond us...the ongoing moment-by-moment interchange between inner and outer...how we breathe out...emptying, trusting that we will be refilled...

Remembering how the breath returns, the life force refilling us again and again...never to be contained or held for long...just moving always in a rhythm that sustains us without our conscious effort...

The Half Moon
Remembering the cycles of the moon...waxing and waning...invisible by day...visible in the dark...

Remembering that I am cyclical too...growing full and visible...retreating into the darkness...

Praying to the Trees
Remembering how the leaves of the oak let go in autumn...how they stand bare...trusting in the slow coming of new growth...how the long needles of the pine stay green and alive beneath the winter snow...

Remembering that we are a part of this...

Praying Up the Sun
Remembering gratitude for the sun on my face from the East...the slow stretching, moving every part of my body...

Remembering my place in relationship with the sun and all that is greater than my little self...

© Rob Angley

SOLO VOICE
Finding Grace by Body Clues

It is not your business to determine how good or
valuable you are, or even to compare yourself with
other artistic forms...your business is to be open.

—*Martha Graham*

In all our lives, there are themes and lessons that we play out over and over. Some of us struggle with feelings of abandonment, fears of rejection, or failure. Others feel victimized or entitled, and some struggle with feeling never good enough. These feelings are often so tender and deep rooted that we learn early on to ignore or negate them. Whatever our life lessons are, they often replay in different forms over and over; in our relationships, at work, with our family, or even in daily interactions with friends or acquaintances. Although individual struggles may vary, the search to understand ourselves through our repeated life lessons and the urge to give form to them through art making is universal.

The lessons I know and struggle with come to me unbidden in numerous guises and arise in many places in my life, and I enact different versions of them in my own relationships, life, and work. Again and again, my deepest lessons have come from the wisdom of my body. They have not always been the lessons I have wanted to hear. At times, they have taken many years to figure out, and other times they have come with both stinging and comforting clarity: My body seems to be saying, "Are you listening, do you get this, do you still need more clues?"

My work, regardless of the medium used in the moment, comes from the grounding and perspective of being a body therapist. Working with the terrain of the body, I often feel as if I am stumbling on unmarked roads, listening for sensation, and waiting for the moment to open. Although I steadfastly believe in the power of verbal therapy, my deepest lessons have come from honoring and acknowledging what my own body already recognizes.

From these realizations, I began to think of our body wisdom like a treasure hunt with many unidentifiable clues along the way. The excerpts that follow come out my work as a body therapist, inspired by a wonderful group that I led several years ago.

Spirit offers a treasure hunt of clues—
mind eclipses our body maps;
our bodies hold the key.

These faint ancient stories
are not written
our bodies draw, not write
all languages dissolve
the symbols, ephemeral legends
can only be gleaned, not held.

Legends are indecipherable
when our body offers
what we are not yet
ready to see.

Although to many onlookers my visceral learning has always come easily, I have always held myself to an almost impossible standard. In relation to other dancers, I have always felt like a slow learner. This is a life struggle that I remember being talked to as a child about, with adults and siblings telling me that my biggest problem was that I had no confidence in myself. Yet as hard as I tried, I felt clearly that I had to define myself by shortcomings, my imperfections; I was always painfully aware that there were so many people better than I! Rationally, I realize that a lack of faith in myself, even in the face of apparent success, has often bound my energy. Physically, I have only recently really admitted to myself that the anxiety I hold within my body disrupts my sense of receptivity and flow. This has been particularly easy to mask because most others see me as loose, fit, and very comfortable in my body. The trap is of trying to be what others see—the perfect therapist!

I came as imposter
pleading, neck exposed
in a body
full of incongruence.

You offered
    marrow stories
maps of courage and pain,
    giggles too.

Humbled by
my stranger within
I took pleasure
in my less than perfect self.

You offered peace
in the most unsettling questions
knowledge that I do not yet understand
I dreamt of unanswerable questions;
your spirits cradled mine.

It was in this state that I received a great lesson: that of surrendering to the circle. There, I could receive the gift of authentic presence that sometimes happens in a cohesive, honest group. I felt undeserving and yet receptive to the love and support that were there, just by being present in the group. And although I was designated as the leader, it was a magical group, one much larger than anyone's own needs, pain, or insecurities. And all my shortcomings or my great moments did not really alter the process of that group. Leader or not, I was not really in charge; we were all just experiencing a state of grace. Whatever my unspoken, interior soundtracks were at the time, I was a privileged witness. Not being in charge was (and is) an uneasy, scary body state for me. But for that moment, I was fed by the group's integrity and courage. I experienced allowing as a life lesson.

In the ocean,
unbound by gravity
whales mate face to face.

In the ocean,
our bodies fly
three dimensionally through space;
There are no maps.
There are only body clues.

Although I, as a teacher and therapist, have felt many successes and moments of "flow" (to use the term that the psychologist Mihaly Csikzentmihalyi [1990] explored in Flow), threads of self-doubt also have permeated my artistic work. At some unconscious level, I long equated being infertile with being uncreative, which physically manifested in a sense of static and anxiety in my body. For years, I felt as if I were dancing exterior shapes, instead of experiencing a felt sense. When choreographing, I had great difficulty trusting the process. I often worked overly hard, to no artistic avail. For some time, I wanted to discard all that came easily to me. I was simply not ready to accept that great progress or choreography or living does not happen by my effort. It has been difficult to reconfigure the discipline-imposed ideals, artistic standards, and expectations that have shaped me as a dancer. My ability to be creative has been eclipsed at times by the pain and fear I did not want to face: that of not being good enough.

Conversely, exploring the arts expressively has allowed me to take joy, to find acceptance in "what is." By immersing myself in poetry, journaling, drawing, and music making, I have no standard to bear. I can easily write, paint, draw, or sing because I expect the process only to produce "what is." "What is" exists without fear of failure or ridicule. I am governed by internal rhythms; I can explore my own fluid, sensual, whimsical pace. Wow—what freedom! I feel like a kid, euphoric with the itch to experiment. My lesson is one of acceptance.

My journey in the expressive arts has brought me full circle, from valuing technical ideals (which are really often based on a model of what isn't) to finding "what is," which exists beyond technique. I have begun to replace unattainable ideals with a picture of the arts as a release, a place of acceptance, a place of grace that does not happen by my effort.

Not by my effort

5 Surgeries
2 Invitro fertilizations
6 Adoptions

Life lessons waiting for me
To be ready to learn

Not by my effort
That's what my body finally said

Waiting for me to hear...
To listen

To stop hammering
Long enough

To feel pain &
Sense wholeness

My bones contain both.

These are integrative moments of life and art. We all have pictures to reformulate about how our lives will be. How we choose to fill in our life pictures shapes how we bring art into life. My life has not had the children I thought I would have. It has been filled with children and connections and family of other sorts.

I have been able to stand and speak with gratitude for a mentor who has touched and shaped hundreds of other lives. I have witnessed my niece, dancing circles on her great-grandmother's grave, throw flower petals and say, "Let's make a ritual." I have seen students soar way beyond their roots and still come back with grateful acknowledgment. I've made dances borne of deep personal pain that later move strangers beyond words...these are moments of bringing life into art, and grace.

—*Marianne Adams*

State of Grace

Old sidewalk unlevel
Sage green grass triumphs through the cracks
Light is changing from day to dusk
I am not big enough to sit and reach the pedals,
too.

No aluminum/titanium parts then—
All heavy metal, big, hard rubber tires
Light years away from gears
Mountain bikes or even banana seats

Sweat and summer's grime on my lips
Wisps of hair, long out of the day's pony tail
Wander across my face
One gnarled hand guides my bike seat
The other guides my handle bar

She lets go—
I falter, panic into tears

She's still there
Her voice brings me out of fear
Back to the present.

"Do you realize that I'm the only one
Who will still help you?"
Tears of frustration well in my eyes

"If you say I can't
One more time,
I won't help anymore
You've got to stop
Thinking you can't
And start trying again."

At that moment,
I feel a terrific push
My grandmother lets go
And her belief in me

Flies me
Into a state of grace.

—Marianne Adams

(see plate #7)

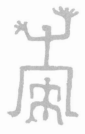

W orking with groups challenges the therapist in a variety of ways. So often, expressive arts experiences are presented simply as activities to be "done" without the necessary preparation, time, and processing for deep emotions to be felt and expressed by group members. Therefore, the primary challenge for the therapist is to be aware of the dynamics of each individual, the dynamics of the group, and ways these dynamics interact with the arts experience in process. Also, the therapist must be sensitive to the flow of the experience—creating a safe space, moving in, working deeply, moving out, and bringing closure. This awareness and sensitivity are what separate the artist-therapist from the activity leader.

Another challenge for the therapist is to know when to intervene and when to remain silent and allow the art to speak for itself. Silence is sacred and often allows a pregnant space for individual processing to occur. It is important that the therapist be comfortable not only with her silence but also with that of others. All too often, words sabotage at critical moments.

The power of making art in the presence of others is not to be underestimated. Emotions that participants experience may range from liberation to rage. It is vital that the therapist not only bear witness to these emotions but be prepared to help the participants stay with and move through emotions evoked by the experience, thereby enhancing growth.

The purpose of this chapter is to present examples of expressive arts experiences that can be facilitated within a group setting. Communal art making is an ancient practice and a privilege to witness. The experiences presented in this chapter can be used to allow communities of people to come together and share in the deeply satisfying endeavor of making art. These experiences reflect parts of the cycle—beginning, moving in, insearch, finding voice, and bringing art into life—and can be adapted in a variety of ways for use in different group settings.

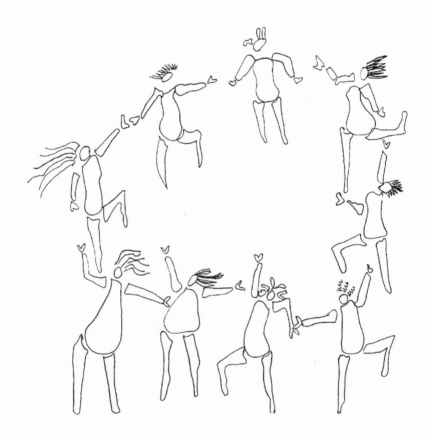

© Genie Gunn

Beginning: Name Improvisation

As a group comes together for the first time, rhythm can be a powerful force to organize, energize, and unite the group members. This simple experience uses the individuals' names to help group members connect with each other, to invite participation in a nonthreatening experience, and to encourage a sense of universality among participants.

1. Begin a "grounding beat," a steady pulse, by gently patting your legs. Invite the group to join.

2. Invite each participant in turn to say his or her first name in whatever rhythm or inflection desired. The group will reflect each name back to the speaker, using the speaker's rhythm and inflection. It may be useful to begin with yourself and then proceed around the circle. Keep the pulse going throughout.

3. On a second round, have each person speak her name in the way her mother called her from outside to come to dinner. The group reflects each one.

4. On a third round, have each person speak his name in the way that his parent called him when he was "in trouble." It may be best not to reflect this one!

5. On a fourth round, have each person speak her name in the way it is spoken by someone who loves her. The group reflects each one.

6. On a final round, each person in turn begins to speak his name in any way he chooses. After he has said it at least three times, the next person adds her name in any rhythm and any inflection she chooses. After she has said her name at least three times, the next person adds his name, and so forth around the circle. Any group member can change how she says her name whenever she wants. Everyone continues until all names are added.

7. To end, there are many options, including these:

    a. Accelerate the grounding beat into a "drum roll," crescendoing to a peak and then signal a cutoff.

    b. Maintaining the pulse, continue around the circle, "layering out" each name in the order it was entered or in random order determined by individual participants.

Moving Inward: Mirroring

This is a well-known exercise in theater that effectively illustrates how people can and do pay attention to one another. This exercise deepens the connections participants experience with each other by means of nonverbal communication.

Divide into pairs. One person is the leader and the other is the follower. The leader will begin with simple arm movements that the follower will mimic in mirror fashion (leader's right hand rises; follower's left hand rises simultaneously, in the same manner, and at the same rate—just as it would in a mirror). As the exercise develops, the leader may use more and more complex movements, employing more of the body; even feet may move but should remain in the same few square feet of floor space. After a time, the pair switches roles. A pair may elect to move without designating a leader to see if they can eliminate leading and following in favor of mutual "attending." Participants can switch partners several times.

Processing of this experience can include a discussion with your most recent partner or a general group discussion. Also, participants can reflect on this experience by creative expression in another medium such as visual art or writing.

Moving In: Drum Circle

Rhythm is everywhere, around us and within us. We experience it with every inhalation and exhalation of the breath, the beat of our hearts, the pulsing of blood through the body, the rhythm of sexual union, the cycles of day and night, the phases of the moon, the seasons of the year. Working with

© Rob Angley

rhythm is a powerful means of tapping into healing forces that are both personal and universal. Effective therapists unconsciously match their breathing with that of their clients.

The ancient instruments of drums and rattles are used by indigenous cultures all over the world for calling in the spirits, for altering states of consciousness, for communicating in community, and for healing. In West Africa the drums do not accompany the dancers; instead, the dancers follow the lead of the drums. Among Native Americans the drumbeat is the heartbeat of Mother Earth. The drum itself represents the union of the plant world, the tree who gave itself for the body of the drum; the animal world, the animal who gave its skin for the head of the drum; and the human being who plays the drum, the person who is privileged to come into that communion.

Because drumming has been practiced in community for centuries and across many cultures, including the West (as with rock and roll bands), it is more universal than some other arts experiences. As a result, drumming may be less threatening than perhaps mask making or dancing and is an ideal experience for "moving in." When structured in a safe manner by the therapist, drumming invites individuals to begin to explore the instrument in their own manner and to later adapt what they play to fit the group. It creates an ideal space for allowing a group to experience the essence of individual rhythm in harmony.

Facilitating Rhythmic Harmony

When you begin a drum circle with a group, teach participants the names of the drums and perhaps give some background information on the instruments, particularly if they are ethnic. Drums hold an honorable place in many cultures, and it is helpful to communicate that respect to participants. Another way to emphasize respect for the instruments is to teach participants some technique for striking the drum either with a mallet or with the hands. (Before offering this experience, you may want to seek training from a professional drummer so you can help the participants play the drums more authentically and, therefore, more satisfyingly.) Once some technique has been presented, allow participants to explore playing the drums on their own.

After participants have gained some confidence through exploring the instruments, bring the group back together and present some simple patterns that everyone can echo. It is important initially to present simple patterns and then move to more complex rhythms.

At some point when participants seem to feel comfortable echoing the patterns, allow participants to make up their own patterns and have the group echo them. Some participants may feel threatened by this experience, so it is helpful to allow participants "to pass" when necessary.

After the drummers are confident with a repertoire of patterns, move into improvisation—an essential part of this experience. Often this transition feels chaotic, and initially the patterns won't seem to fit; however, this is a natural process that occurs when groups attempt to improvise. At this point it is critical that you sit with the chaos.

Somehow the muses always enter, and miraculously the individual patterns will find their way into rhythmic harmony. This moment is the essence of the drum circle, where all are hearing how their individual music is supported by and integrated into that of the other performers, a beautiful metaphor for further processing.

End the improvisation with some signal to the group, or allow the piece to find its way into closure. Once the piece has ended, help participants explore and articulate their emotions associated with the experience of music making within a group.

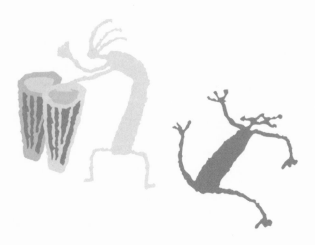

INSEARCH: SOLITUDE

The place of insearch is deep and personal and solitary. It is the place where we find paradox, both shadows and deep truth. This is a place of solitude, but there is a wonderful paradox of finding an experience of deep inner stillness alone, while at the same time being in the company of others with a similar intention.

Alone Time for Group Members

Ask each participant to spend one hour (or one day) alone in the natural world, not writing, not speaking with anyone or "doing" anything, but simply paying attention to both inner and outer experiences. Spending time alone is the essence of this exercise. Being in the natural world is suggested because of the rich possibilities of experiencing ourselves as a small part of the whole of the natural world. For some, even the stimulation of being outside can be a distraction from inner awareness.

In our world, the experience of alone time is often difficult for many people. Accustomed to the constant bombardment of information, sound, and image of our fast-paced technological society, it is rare for most of us to spend even one hour alone and not engaged in activity. Simply holding space in this way often allows for deep immersion into the realm of the creative, the place of the shadow, the place of paradox.

Three Modalities for Processing

The experience of alone time can be explored through a variety of modalities. Each modality has its own laws of form, which suggest multileveled metaphors and provoke different questions. Each one can be used separately, or they can be used together for a layered experience. Three modalities that offer rich possibilities for processing are (a) writing, (b) clay, and (c) collage.

Writing. Allow time (thirty to forty-five minutes) immediately following the solitude experience for participants to reflect upon the experience in free writing. That is, participants should be encouraged simply to accept whatever comes and to record it. This provides the opportunity for naming the experience and exploring its meaning in words. Such writing often reveals unexpected surprises.

Clay. Following the solitude experience, each participant is offered the opportunity to work with clay (forty-five minutes to one hour). Literally working with earth has a powerful grounding and centering effect. Once again, each participant should be encouraged to relax and to let the clay shape itself. The use of instrumental music while participants remain silent can further deepen the experience. Images from the unconscious, symbols of aspects of the self and of life, often emerge in this way.

Collage. Creating a visual artpiece that is an assemblage of images cut and pasted from magazines is another form of creative processing of an experience of solitude. This modality affords access to a wide and sophisticated array of images, words, shapes, and colors, even for a person with no training or experience in visual art-making. This activity requires a large block of time (one to three hours). This modality suggests metaphors of layers and of pieces of a whole.

Group Sharing

It is important to close this experience with some group sharing, but this can be very brief. For written responses, the sharing could be structured by having each participant complete the sentence I experienced...For artwork, the sharing might simply involve participants showing and titling their work.

Finding Voice: Visual Self-expression

Mark making is one of the primary means by which we express our subjective issues and concerns. Our tools (brushes, pencils, pens, etc.) usually come with expected, or predicted, marking characteristics, but it is the unique muscular responses of the artist that personalize even the most common of marking tools.

One compelling example comes from an art class I conducted at a summer church camp. When one of the children in the class complained about being homesick, several other campers voiced similar feelings, and we talked for a few minutes about homesickness and feelings such as fear, joy, and sadness. Acting more on instinct than experience, I asked each of them to take their tempera paint and visualize some of these emotional states. "Try," I said, "to convey homesickness with your brush." At first, some of the children tried to create symbols to represent the source of their homesickness (symbols of their mothers, their dogs, etc.), but as they got more comfortable with the exercise, they realized they did not need to employ symbols to express their feelings. They found that the marks, themselves, could convey their emotions.

One nine-year-old boy drew this:

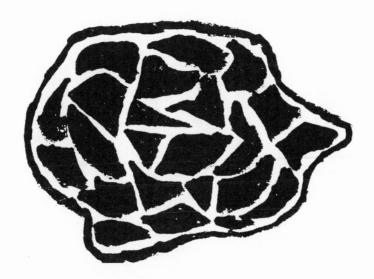

Later, when we talked about our drawings, he said:

Ever since I can remember, my mother and father sent me to summer camp so they could travel in Europe. I have been homesick many times, and I have cried a lot. The small, jagged shapes are my tears, but I have tied them up so my mother and father cannot see them. They would be angry if they were to see this drawing.

This young boy realized that it was through his empathy with the sensation of homesickness that he was able to express his painful feelings.

Self-expression in Mark Making

To explore mark making with a group, have the group members collect and bring to this experience an assortment of found materials. Allow them to explore the marking response made by each of these objects by dipping the object in ink and then depositing the ink to the page. This is not about drawing anything...this is about marking. Encourage play with the materials, exploring various ways of depositing ink onto the paper. Here are a few examples.

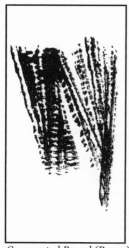
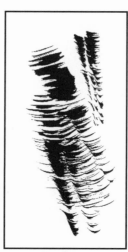
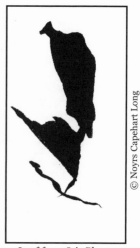

Corrugated Board (Paper)   *Feather*   *Leaf from Iris Plant*

Have each participant select five or six favorite markings. Starting with a clean piece of newsprint paper, explore the markings further. Experiment with the found objects and notice the images that develop.

Next, have the participants select an emotional theme such as one of the following:

nausea
jealousy
envy
anger
surprise
ecstasy

Encourage members of the group to empathize with their theme. Suggest that participants allow their feelings and connection with the theme to dictate their marking rhythms. Urge the participants to "feel" their way through this experience—without any predetermined solutions or symbols to represent tangible objects. Allow participants to create two or three responses to the same theme, reminding participants that first responses are not always going to yield their strongest response.

Finally, have participants hang selected images around the room. Invite members of the group to respond to the images that draw their attention and appeal to them most strongly. Also allow participants to share and discuss the emotional theme portrayed in their images.

—Contributed by Noyes Capehart Long and adapted by Scarlet Tison

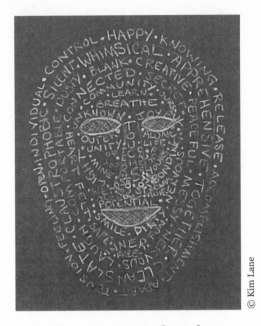

© Kim Lane

Finding Voice: Mask Making

Masks have been used for hundred of years in diverse cultures all over the world. Most often they have been used in spiritual and social rituals to represent spirit powers or archetypal forms to celebrate seasonal cycles, to affirm the union of human beings with the natural world, to honor stages of human development, to pray for success in hunts and harvests, and to provide guidelines for human actions.

Ancient cave paintings show hunting scenes with masked dancers. Greek masks were used in a variety of rituals, and later actors in theatrical productions adopted masks to indicate tragic, comic, or satiric characters. The Medieval church used masks in mystery plays all over Europe. Masks appear in the entire history of China, as early as the Chou dynasty, when bronze masks were used. Masks or painted faces are typical in Chinese theater. Over one hundred varieties of masks are used in the No dramas of Japan, to represent human beings, gods, demons, and animals. Australian aboriginal tribes and the tribes of western and central Africa all used masks or face painting.

In both North and South America masks are used in ceremonies and in secret societies. The Hopi and Zuni kachinas are examples of the use of masks by the Pueblo tribes of the American Southwest. The masked societies of the Iroquois have survived for over three centuries. The most important of them, the "False Face Society," is a medicine society concerned with the curing of illnesses. As in most primitive masked societies the wearing of the mask makes one psychically identical with the supernatural being represented.

Masks are used to express our human need for transcendence and to fulfill our fundamental longing for the mysterious. Masks both hide and reveal. They hide the identity of the person who wears the mask, and they reveal some universal aspect that is larger than the individual.

Creating masks is a way of giving form to an inner truth. Deep involvement means that the work itself becomes more important than the self-consciousness of the artist. It is important to honor the authentic creative act.

Group Process with Mask Making

Through the process of creating and sharing masks, group members can explore such questions as

- How do we hide ourselves?
- How do we reveal the truth of who we are?
- How do we invite the larger forces of spirit and the natural world to be expressed through us?
- How do we use these powers in service of growth and healing in our lives?

Constructing the Mask

Materials

- Plaster bandage—approximately one three-inch roll per person, cut into strips of varying sizes
- Scissors
- Petroleum jelly
- Scarf or bandana to tie back hair
- Towel and washcloth
- Container for water for dipping bandage

Have participants work in groups of three and take turns building a plaster mask on each person. Compassion, self-protection, and comfort are important facets of this process. The person whose mask is being constructed must tie back her hair and cover the face completely with petroleum jelly. She then lies down in a comfortable place with eyes closed and with a towel protecting the area around the face. The rest of the group then works together to construct the mask. Larger pieces of bandage provide structural support, and smaller pieces are used to shape the contours. Three or four layers of material are sufficient. Generally, eyes and nostrils are not covered. Play some relaxing music during this process. Attention and intention deepen the process. Following completion of all the masks, ask the participants to reflect on the experience. (Allow three to four hours for this phase.)

Decorating the Mask

After the masks have dried completely (approximately one week later), have the participants decorate their masks, using paint, glue, and any other materials available, such as yarn, feathers, fur, leather, beads, and natural objects. It is important for you to provide a wide variety of materials. You may suggest themes, such as animal spirit guides, the shadow side of the personality, or parts of the self, but most often it is best to encourage the participants to enter a relaxed state and let forms emerge uncensored. (Allow three to four hours for this phase.) This phase may be done individually at home, but it is an opportunity for group building as people work together and pool resources.

Presenting the Mask

After the masks have been finished, have participants present themselves in their masks to each other in dance, music, story, or other dramatic form. Allow time for responses to each participant and for general sharing. (This can be done in a very abbreviated form with one to two minutes for highly structured sharing or in a more in-depth way by allowing ten to fifteen minutes per person for sharing.)

Clinical Applications

This activity is appropriate for a group that has developed a high level of trust, for several reasons. First, part of the purpose of this activity is to see and reveal ourselves in ways that mirrors or photographs do not allow. Also, trust and respect must be firmly established prior to working so intimately with another's face. In our culture, oftentimes, touching another's face is a privilege given only to those closest to us. This may be a boundary you can explore before starting the activity, to decrease participants' anxiety and apprehension regarding physical contact.

Mask making may be used with people who have identity issues or addictions, have experienced trauma, or are working on personal growth and identity strengthening. A mask can enable someone to explore an unexpected identity. It can act as a window to the soul.

—Contributed by Toni Carlton, Mary Beth Rabon, and Sally Atkins

(See Plate #8.)

Entering the Mask

Hollow and weak out
of his fast, he bore the mask
to his face. Large horns,
incurving flaming arrow
rising from the third eye up
the brow like the prow
of a ship set sail. Scars
like waves on either
side. The yonder shore
in ebony—hard wood,
hard, hard wood—
shelling the skin against
hard stares of children
and the fire he was about
to enter that would enter
him, to chart the course, tie
and untie, furl and unfurl
sheets in wind and steer
his course. An ancient
voice rose in him deeper
than drum or chant
breathing down to bone,
hurling him against
the night filled with fire
and the darker for it. All
light was from the glow
of his own skin fueled
by the oil of his heart.
As in a dance, he
advanced over North Peak
where he felt the voice
conjure magnificent beasts
wreathed in snow, hung
with ice and thunder.
Down to the savannah
through the tales whispered
in tall grass and choked
by the pattern of cracked mud.
West Mountain, he saw, was
built of bones whose dry
sharp clicking was like his own
language spoken by a
stranger.

The cave of South Range
swallowed him, spun him
like the ancestor who first
made love to the earth
when she was a girl. He
could neither see nor stand,
just fall and let himself fall.
East Mountain opened
to him the dream of home
and journey's end, as
always his people had
known return, shaped
by One whose slide
down its side left
laughter in the odor
of its flowers, but laughter
left him as he rode wind's
leopard scream straight
into the sun, black and
blazing.
Blind and overcome
by the sun's aroma
he tore a piece with his teeth.
Hot fat melted his fear
and filled his heart even
as stars died and waves—
dashed upon familiar ground—
crept back upon his face
which then replaced hard
wood, its power dissolved
as strength ran like sand
from his legs, replaced
by tears of hunger for his
his children and wife
of twenty years. This man
who hardly recognized
himself and now recognized
himself too well.

—Jay Wentworth

Bringing Art into Life: Makwa

In West Africa, there is a type of handclapping that occurs spontaneously and is improvised to accompany dance or just to make music. Makwa is rarely accompanied by other percussive instruments. The beauty of Makwa is that each person performs a different rhythm pattern, and they all come together to create a beautiful and complex piece. The metaphor is obvious: each of us must individuate before rejoining others in a community to make "music." The foundation for real music making is when many complex ideas come together to create harmony. What a beautiful metaphor for accepting the diversity of each human and recognizing the potential for a harmonious community.

Creating Community through Rhythms

This exercise can be a metaphor for moving from a place of the inner self back into the outside world, bringing a new and unique voice back into community.

- Break up your group into five smaller groups.
- Establish eight steady beats on a drum.
- Teach each group by rote one pattern, and have them practice the pattern within their groups. For example, for pattern 1, the group would only clap on beats 1, 3, 5, and 6.

1	2	3	4	5	6	7	8
X		X		X	X		
X			X			X	
	X				X		X
	X	X			X	X	
X	X	X		X		X	

- When the group members seem comfortable, ask them to move out within the group, find one person with a different pattern, and clap those patterns simultaneously. Eventually, encourage the entire group to walk around and clap their patterns while noticing how other patterns complement theirs. Also encourage everyone to listen carefully to the beauty of the "whole" piece.

Bringing Art into Life: Creating Maps

An introduction to maps is described by the physicist David Peat in his 1991 book, *The Philosopher's Stone: Chaos, Synchronicity, and the Hidden Order of the World.* He begins with the observation that we, as humans, seek to understand our experiences in the world. In doing so, we create images and symbols that serve to connect the outer, physical world with our personal, inner experiences. A map is a symbolic representation of the relationship between the external and internal events. Peat writes, "Maps, symbols, mandalas, petroglyphs, and other symbolic works are used all over the world to express the link between the inner and outer, between the self and the world, the individual and the environment. Such maps enrich us and bind us together" (p. 14).

A simple road map is an example familiar to those in Western societies. It is a symbolic guide to aspects of the physical world (using direction, measured distance, location in space) that reflect the personal experience of moving from place to place. This kind of map is familiar because it describes how we often think and feel about moving around in our environment. A map designed by Australian Aboriginal people, however, taps a very different relationship between inner and outer experience and uses very different symbols. For example, units of direction and distance are secondary to the spiritual and creative events that define a "place" for them. A map identifying a significant, sacred place may contain images of human and animal footprints, spiral landscapes (rivers, mountains), colors, textures, and songs that connect individuals to their ancestors and to the origins of creation in the Dreamtime. Aboriginal maps may seem strange because they reflect a way of experiencing the world that is very different from our own (Peat, 1991).

Invite each member of your group to create a map that in some way reveals a connection between his own experiences and aspects of the outer world. The map does not necessarily have to be two-dimensional or drawn on paper; it can express symbolically any aspects of inner and outer life in relation to each other. After the maps are completed, ask the participants to provide some verbal and/or written descriptions of or stories about their maps and what those mean to them. The following map and its description were contributed by Brooke Cranswick, a student in a college honors class on human culture and boundaries.

Description: My map is a picture of me, of my current life-journey through the time continuum. Time is infinite (as far as is known) and we see time only in small intervals. One visual manifestation of time is that of the spiral—quite similar to the general infinity symbol. A "cross-section" of that representation is what my map signifies, the cross-section of my existence, of the existence of the everlasting components of the universe put in my personal order. What we see on the paper is all events of my past, from birth to present date, all that I can remember being a part of me. In essence, the map is a chronological representation of all influential events in the making of me. The invisible line spiraling from the center to the outer circle is what I consider the "norm." The curls and loops symbolize my experiences as Brooke, the unusual or unexpected or important or enlightening times in my life. Should I have never deviated from what is "right," my map would be thin and boring, following a circular yet horribly linear lifeline. Each bulge has a meaning, and can symbolize a rite of passage, a realization, a common sense lesson, a first breath, or one of many other events. I envisioned the dotted lines to be a subconscious knowledge of self, not yet unleashed to the world. Loops and swirls delineate times of confusion and ignorance and regression, while more straight lines are symbolic of times of awareness and intelligence and self-knowledge. Most of the meaning of the map remains unknown to me in my humane ignorance, and is a subconscious outpouring of what I felt needed to be represented at the time of creation. A very important concept of the map cannot be forgotten: that it is infinite. The spiral goes inward and outward and appears to stop at the ends of the circle's radius. In this map, the spiral continues into that which we cannot see: forever. This map is only a teeny tiny bit of the infinite existence (that matter which cannot be created or destroyed) that surrounds and comprises us.

© Brooke Cranswick

—*Contributed by Joan Woodworth*

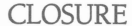

CLOSURE

The work of making this book has been an experiment in interdisciplinary collaboration in expressive arts. We have participated in every cycle of the creative process that we have described. We have shared our beginning, our daily practices, our fears and resistance, and our sources of inspiration. Together, we have moved into creative space and sought the wisdom that enabled us to taste shadow and touch light. We have given voice to our personal experience and our collective wisdom, and we have sought to bring our learnings from expressive arts into our lives.

This has not been easy work. At every stage this work has been about prizing differences and owning both strengths and weaknesses. Again and again the work has demanded that we deepen our own process, individually and collectively, to speak our own truths clearly and openly. Time and again the work has called for us to let go of individual ego in service of the collective goal and to trust the process.

We are reminded of the eternal cycles of creative process of which our work together is a small part. We remember the cycles of breath, cycles of days and moons and seasons, cycles of individuals and groups, and the cycles of the human story.

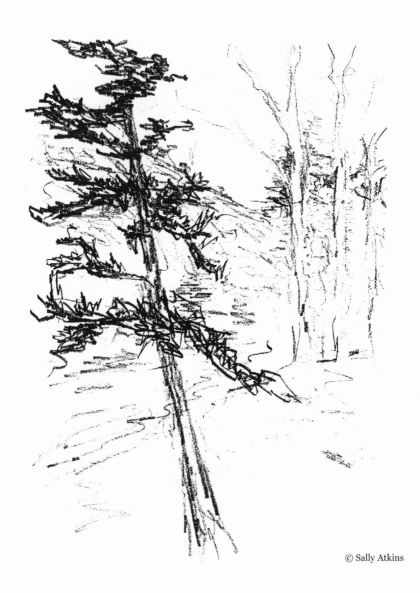

© Sally Atkins

Cycle

We sit in the circle silently. Words become our invocation:
> *Be still...*
> *Wherever you are is called here...*

We go around, sunwise,
Casting the circle with our words to each other.
Today this is where I am, this is who I am.
Each one of us speaks into this circle
Weaving ourselves together in this holy space,
Acknowledging the interconnectedness that already is.

We speak of safety,
How to make a place that is safe
For work that is personal and deep,
Work that is beautiful...and not always pretty,
A place that is safe to be all of who we are.
We speak of honesty, integrity,
How to stand to the truth of our whole selves.
We speak of intention, of commitment
To our own and each other's learning and growth.

We speak of bearing witness,
What it means to hold the space,
To be present to another's work.
We claim the language of feeling and emotion,
The language of the body.
We name:
> *courage   fear   longing   excitement   pain   joy*
And we let them move in our bodies.

Something happens.
There is no lesson plan, but there are many lessons.
There are ideas, information, experiences, and reflection.
This is a dance of the mind, and we are all the choreographers.
This is a dance of the body, we are alive, breathing, now.
This is a dance of spirit, something greater
Than our little skin-encapsulated selves is moving among us.

We are alive, learning,
      from teachers, from books,
      from each other, from ourselves,
      from some place of wisdom, ancient and deep.

We close with silence, joining hands to remember
There are words of blessing:
      Walk carefully, well-loved ones.

The candle is extinguished.
The circle is open but unbroken.

—*Sally Atkins*

CONTRIBUTORS' NOTES

Appalachian Expressive Arts Collective Members

Marianne Adams holds a master of fine arts degree in dance and a master's degree in clinical psychology. She is currently integrating these two fields through her work as a professor at Appalachian State University. She has received numerous grants in support of her work as a dancer and choreographer, including a 1987 NC Choreographer's Fellowship. Marianne has also worked as a therapeutic movement specialist in several mental health settings. She has been a certified Pilates instructor since 1998. She is a founding member of the Appalachian Expressive Arts Collective and greatly enjoys participating in collaborative art making, teaching, and therapy.

Sally Atkins holds master's and doctoral degrees in counseling. She is a licensed psychologist and a registered expressive arts therapist. She is a professor in the Department of Human Development and Psychological Counseling, and a faculty/staff psychologist at the Hubbard Center at Appalachian State University. She has been a practicing psychotherapist for twenty-seven years and is a member of the American Academy of Psychotherapists. Her teaching and research interests include therapy and the arts, cross-cultural healing practices, and consciousness and dreamwork. In 1999 she received the North Carolina Board of Governors Award for Outstanding Teaching. She is a storyteller, ritualist, dancer, and poet. Sally is a founding member of the Appalachian Expressive Arts Collective.

Cathy McKinney has a doctoral degree in music therapy and behavioral medicine and a master's degree in music therapy. A board-certified music therapist with twenty years' clinical experience in a variety of settings, she is currently serving as an associate professor and the director of music therapy at Appalachian State University. Her current clinical interests are the use of music improvisation and the Bonny Method of Guided Imagery and Music as vehicles for personal awareness, growth, and transformation. A Fellow of the Association for Music and Imagery, Cathy is a founding member of the Appalachian Expressive Arts Collective.

Harold McKinney holds doctoral and master's degrees in music. He is a certified teacher of Creative Motion and teaches annually at the Creative Motion Alliance's Windswept Music Workshop in Kansas City, Missouri. He has led sessions on Creative Motion and Personal Growth, as well as dream workshops, throughout the United States. Harold currently serves as a professor of music at Appalachian State University, where he teaches applied music and an experiential graduate course in philosophy of music. He is a founding member of the Appalachian Expressive Arts Collective.

Liz Rose is a board-certified music therapist and has a doctoral degree in music education. She is an associate professor of music education and therapy at Appalachian State University. Liz is certified in Dalcroze Eurhythmics, a methodology that emphasizes coming to know music through expressive movement, and she has presented clinics nationally. Liz has worked as a music therapist and educator in a variety of clinical and public school settings. Her professional interests include creativity and the arts, as well as expressive musicianship through Dalcroze Eurhythmics.

Jay Wentworth holds a doctorate in dramatic literature and degrees in philosophy, theology and culture, and English, as well as a postgraduate certificate from the Gestalt Institute of Cleveland. Currently, a professor in interdisciplinary studies at Appalachian State University, he is on the Board of Directors of the Association for Integrative Studies and edits the association's journal, *Issues in Integrative Studies*. He has been a senior staff, lay psychotherapist at The Country Place in Litchfield, Connecticut. He is a published poet who has also written two opera librettos and has collaborated with the Broyhill Chamber Ensemble on several performances as a writer and performer. The Atlanta Ballet Company has accepted his children's story "The Tree of Fallen Stars" as the basis for a ballet.

Joan Woodworth holds a doctorate in psychology with a concentration in the history of science. Currently a professor of psychology at Appalachian State University, she teaches courses in history and systems and integrative paradigms in psychology. Her professional interests include the cross-cultural study of dreams, consciousness studies, and ecopsychology.

❀ ❀ ❀ ❀ ❀

Terri Chester, a former member of the Appalachian Expressive Arts Collective, has a master's degree in agency counseling. She is a licensed professional counselor, a national certified counselor, and a licensed school counselor in North Carolina. She has been working as a teacher and counselor for eighteen years in various settings, including private practice, public school, mental health, university, and community college ones. Terri is a doctoral candidate in expressive arts therapies at the European Graduate School in Switzerland. She was a founding member of the Expressive Arts Collective.

Expressive Arts Therapy Editor

Sharon A. Sharp, an editor and a poet, holds doctoral and master's degrees in human development and family studies, as well as a bachelor's degree in English. She has edited more than ninety books for publishers such as HarperCollins, Addison-Wesley, and Kodansha, and has focused on trade nonfiction books related to health, psychology, social issues, and education. She has also edited scholarly journal articles, conference proceedings, newsletters, special reports, and other materials. She has taught human development, family studies, and sociology at the college level, and for the past eight years has taught editing in the Department of English at Appalachian State University. She currently serves as the president of the North Carolina Poetry Society and as a member of the North Carolina Writers' Network, the North Carolina Writers Conference, and the National Association for Poetry Therapy. Author of the chapbook *Personal Effects*, she has also had numerous poems published in literary magazines.

Other Expressive Arts Therapy Contributors and Source Acknowledgments

The Expressive Arts Collective members gratefully acknowledge contributions by the following people, who granted permission for their works to be included in this book and who remain the copyright holders. Some of these works also appeared in the Expressive Arts Collective's earlier books, *Expressive Arts: An Invitation to the Journey and Collective Voices in Expressive Arts* (Hubbard Center for Faculty and Staff Support, Appalachian State University).

Articles

Marianne Adams: A revised version of "Finding Grace by Body Clues" (pp. 116-121) has appeared in the *Journal of Poetry Therapy;* it is reprinted with permission of the publisher.

Sally Atkins: Portions of "Becoming an Artist-Therapist" (pp. 18-23) appeared first in *Poiesis: A Journal of the Arts & Communication* and are reprinted with permission of the publisher.

Toni Carlton: Portions of "Finding Voice: Mask Making" (pp. 134-136).

Noyes Capehart Long: "Finding Voice: Visual Self-Expression" as adapted by Scarlet Tison (pp. 131-133).

Mary Beth Rabon: Portions of "Finding Voice: Mask Making" (pp. 134-136).

Artwork

Rob Angley: Drawings (pp. 115 and 126).

Laurie Atkins: Pencil drawing (p. 64).

Ty Atkins: Graphic design (p. 98).

Bingham Dai: "Tao" (p. 70) and "Ren" (p. 87).

Brooke Cranswick: Personal map and description (p. 140).

Lori Fowler-Hill: *St. John's Wort* (p. 39), untitled pencil drawing (p. 51), untitled pencil drawing (p. 68), and *Passing Down the Wisdom* (p. 110).

Genie Gunn: Pen and ink drawing (p. 124).

Patience Harrison: Drawing within Jill Masten-Byers's "Being in the Creative" (p. 75).

Kim Lane: Pencil drawing (p. 134).

Noyes Capehart Long: Three ink images (p. 132) are used by permission of the artist-author.

Sybil Metz: Watercolor painting (p. 33).

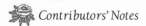

Rhonda Peterson: Drawing (p. 62).

Liza Shaw: "Spirit Guide" drawing and dream description (p. 69).

Color Plates

Toni Carlton: *Spirit Shield* (Plate #8).

Lori Fowler-Hill: *Home on Fire* (Plate #2), *Demeter* (Plate #3), *Together Not Broken* (Plate #4), *Get Back, no. 1* (Plate #5), and *Union* (Plate #6).

Lindley C. Sharp: Untitled (Plate #1).

Wang Yanbin: Untitled (Plate #7).

Poetry

Marianne Adams: "Daily Practice" (p. 29), "Mindfulness" (p. 66), "Tasting Shadows Touching Light" (p. 70), "It Helps to Remember" (p. 115), "Not By My Effort" (p. 124), "State of Grace" (p. 125).

Terri Chester: "Centering" (p. 35), "Fears" (p. 57), "The Race" (p. 57), "Prayer for Angels" (p. 105).

Cathy McKinney: "Wellspring" (p. 31), "Woman on a Rack" (p. 111).

Harold McKinney: "A Story" (p. 111).

Jay Wentworth: "Apple Walk" (p. 63), "On a Hillside: A Dragon's Breath" (p. 107), "Entering the Mask" (p. 142).

Sally Atkins: "Tell Me, She Said" (p. 20) first appeared in *Voices: The Art and Science of Psychotherapy*; it is reprinted by permission of the publisher. "Chaos Theory" (p. 22) first appeared in *Poiesis: A Journal of the Arts & Communication*.

Kate Brinko: "Wrightsville Beach" (p. 48).

Kirtan Coan: "Cold at the Poet's Fire" (p. 55), "Tenderness and Dignity" (p. 63), and "Just Drink" (p. 99).

Catherine Cope: "Misknowmer" (p. 79).

Mark Larsen: "Poem Drum" (p. 79).

Jill Masten-Byers: "Dancing can be anything" (p. 42) and "Being in the Creative" (p. 75).

Pam Noble: "Heart's Intention" (p. 114).

Sharon A. Sharp: "Yoga Embrace" (p. 39) first appeared in Southern Dharma Retreat Center Newsletter; "Refuge" (p. 50), in the Journal of Poetry Therapy; and "Centersearch" (p. 76), in Writing Our Lives. These are reprinted by permission of the poet, with thanks to the publishers. Other poems: "Awakening" (p. 45), "Freehand" (p. 93), and "Recognition" (p. 105).

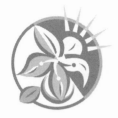

BIBLIOGRAPHY

Creativity/Personal Growth

Artress, L. (1995). *Walking a sacred path: Rediscovering the labyrinth as a spiritual tool.* New York: Riverhead.

Arieti, S. (1976). *Creativity: The magic synthesis.* New York: Basic Books.

de Avila, T. (1980). *The collected works of St. Teresa of Avila, Vol. II.* (K. Kavanaugh & O. Rodriquez, Trans.). Washington, DC: ICS. (Original work published 1566.)

Baird, P. *The pyramid cookbook.* New York: Henry Holt.

Bender, S. (1995). *Everyday sacred.* San Fransisco: HarperSanFransisco.

Breathnach, S. B. (1995). *Simple abundance: A daybook of comfort and joy.* New York: Warner Books.

Cameron, J. (1992). *The artist's way.* New York: Tarcher/Perigee.

Cameron, J. (1996). *The vein of gold.* New York: Tarcher/Putnam.

Cameron, J., Goldberg, N., Metzger, D., Jarret, K., Allende, I., & Csikszentmihalyi, M. (1997). *The well of creativity.* Carlsbad, CA: Hay House.

Ganim, B. (1999). *Art and healing.* New York: Three Rivers.

Lightman, A. (1993). *Einstein's dreams.* New York: Warner Books.

Lightman, A. (1996). *Dance for two.* New York: Pantheon Books.

Lyden, S. C. (1997). *The knitting sutra: Craft as a spiritual practice.* San Francisco: HarperSanFrancisco.

Margulies, A. (1989). *The empathic imagination.* New York: Norton.

Moustakas, C. (1967). *Creativity and conformity.* New York: Van Nostrand.

Nachmanovitch, S. (1990). *Free play: Creativity in life and art.* New York: Tarcher/Perigee.

Pearson, C. (1989). *The hero within: Six archetypes we live by.* San Francisco: Harper & Row.

Richards, M. C. (1966). *The crossing point.* Middletown, CT: Wesleyan University Press.

Richards, M. C. (1989). *Centering: In poetry, pottery, and the person* (2nd ed.). Middletown, CT: Wesleyan University Press.

Richards, M. C. (1996). *Opening our moral eye: Essays, talks, and poems embracing creativity and community.* Hudson, NY: Lindisfarne Press.

Robbins, A. (1985). *Waking up in the age of creativity.* Santa Fe, NM: Bear.

Samuels, M., & Lane, M. R. (1998). *Creative healing.* San Francisco: HarperSanFrancisco.

Staude, J. R. (Ed.). (1977). *Consciousness and creativity.* Berkeley, CA: Ross.

Swimme, B. (1985). *The universe is a green dragon.* Santa Fe, NM: Bear.

Vaughan, F. E. (1979). *Awakening intuition.* Garden City, NY: Anchor/Doubleday.

Walker, A. (1997). *Anything we love can be saved.* New York: Random House.

Wilmer, H. A. (Ed.). (1991). *Creativity: Paradoxes and reflections.* Wilmette, IL: Chiron.

Winterson., J. (1996). *Art (objects): Essays on ecstasy and effrontery.* New York: Knopf.

Expressive Arts Therapy

Allen, P. B. (1995). *Art is a way of knowing.* Boston: Shambhala.

Feder, E., & Feder, B. (1981). *The expressive arts therapies.* Englewood Cliffs, NJ: Prentice Hall.

Knill, P. J., Barba, H. N., & Fuchs, M. N. (1995). *Minstrels of soul: Intermodal expressive therapy.* Toronto, Canada: Palmerston Press.

Levine, E. (1995). *Tending the fire: Studies in art, therapy, and creativity.* Toronto, Canada: Palmerston Press.

Levine, S. K. (1992). Poieses: *The language of psychology and the speech of the soul.* Philadelphia: Kingsley.

Levine, S. K., & Levine, E. G. (1998*). Foundations of expressive arts therapies: Theoretical and classical perspectives.* Philadelphia: Kingsley.

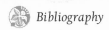

McNiff, S. (1981). *The arts and psychotherapy.* Springfield, IL: Thomas.

McNiff, S. (1986). *Educating the creative arts therapist.* Springfield, IL: Thomas.

McNiff, S. (1992). *Art as medicine: Creating a therapy of the imagination.* Boston: Shambhala.

McNiff, S. (1998). *Art-based research.* Philadelphia: Kingsley.

McNiff, S. (1998). *Trust the process: An artist's guide to letting go.* Boston: Shambhala.

Robbins, A. (1986). *Expressive therapy.* New York: Human Sciences Press.

Rogers, N. (1993). *The creative connection: Expressive arts as healing.* Palo Alto, CA: Science & Behavior Books.

Warren, B. (Ed.). (1984). *Using the creative arts in therapy.* Cambridge, MA: Brookline Books.

Weiss, J. C. (1984). *Expressive therapy with elders and the disabled: Touching the heart of life.* NY: Haworth.

Counseling and Psychological Foundations of Expressive Arts Therapy

von Bertalanffy, L. (1968). *General systems theory: Foundations, development, applications.* New York: Braziller.

Bowen, M. (1978). *Family therapy in clinical practice.* New York: Jason Aronson.

Bugental, J. F. T. (1987). *The art of the psychotherapist.* New York: Norton.

Campbell, J. (1971). *The portable Jung.* New York: Viking.

Capra, F. (1996). *The web of life.* New York: Anchor.

Dallett, J. O. (1988). *When the spirits come back.* Toronto: Inner City.

Freud, S. (1961). An outline of psychoanalysis. In J. Strachey (Ed. and Trans.) *The standard edition of the complete psychological works of Sigmund Freud* (Vol. 23). London: Hogarth Press. (Original work published 1940)

Gladding, S. T. (1998). *Counseling as an art: The creative arts in counseling* (2nd ed.). Alexandria, VA: American Counseling Association.

Harman, W. (1994). Toward a "science of wholeness." In W. Harman & J. Clark (Eds.), *New metaphysical foundations of modern science.* Sausalito, CA: Institute of Noetic Sciences.

Jung, C. (1968). *Analytical psychology: Its theory and practice.* New York: Pantheon.

Jung, C., Von Franz, M. L., Henderson, J. L., Jacobi, J., & Jaffe, R. (1964). *Man and his symbols.* Garden City, NY: Doubleday.

Keyes, M. F. (1983). *Inward journey: Art as therapy.* La Salle, IL: Open Court.

Kuhn, T. (1970). *The structure of scientific revolutions.* Chicago: University of Chicago Press.

Maslow, A. (1962). *Toward a psychology of being.* Princeton: Van Nostrand.

Maslow, A. (1971). *The farther reaches of human nature.* New York: Viking.

May, R. (1975). *The courage to create.* New York: Norton.

Minuchin, S. (1974). *Families and family therapy.* Cambridge, MA: Harvard University Press.

Peat, D. (1991). *The philosopher's stone.* New York: Bantam.

Perls, F. (1973). *The Gestalt approach and eyewitness to therapy.* New York: Bantam.

Satir, V. (1972). *Peoplemaking.* Palo Alto, CA: Science & Behavior.

Sullivan, H. S. (1953). *The interpersonal theory of psychiatry.* New York: Norton.

Tarnas, R. (1991). *The passion of the Western mind.* New York: Harmony.

Wolpe, J. (1958). *Psychotherapy by reciprocal inhibition.* Stanford, CA: Stanford University Press.

Whitaker, C. A. & Bumberry, W. M. (1988*). Dancing with a family: A symbolic-experiential approach.* New York: Brunner/Mazel.

Zinker, J. (1978). *The creative process in Gestalt therapy.* New York: Vintage.

Dance/Movement Therapy

Bartal, L., & Ne'eman, N. (1993). *The metaphoric body: Guide to expressive therapies through images and archetypes.* Bristol, PA: Taylor & Francis.

Bernstein, P. L. (1972). *Theory and methods in dance movement therapy: A manual for therapists, students and educators.* Dubuque, IA: Kendall Hunt.

Blom, L. A., & Chaplin, L. T. (1983). *The intimate act of choreography.* Pittsburgh, PA: University of Pittsburgh Press.

Blom, L. A., & Chaplin, L. T. (1988). *The moment of movement: Dance improvisation.* Pittsburgh, PA: University of Pittsburgh Press.

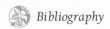

Caplow-Lindner, E. (1979). *Therapeutic dance/movement: Expressive activities for older adults.* New York: Human Sciences Press.

Chodorow, J. (1991). *Dance therapy and depth psychology: The moving imagination.* New York: Routledge.

Cornfield, R. (Ed.). (1998). *Dance, writings, and poetry.* New Haven, CT: Yale University Press.

Friedman, P., & Eisen, G. (1980). *The Pilates method of physical and mental conditioning.* New York: Doubleday.

Gallagher, S. P., & Kryzanowska, R. (1999). *The Pilates method of body conditioning.* Philadelphia: Bainbridge.

Halprin, A. (1995). *Moving toward life: Five decades of transformational dance.* London: Wesleyan University Press.

Highwater, J. (1992). *Dance: Rituals of experience* (3rd ed.). New York: Oxford University Press.

Huang, C. A., & Lynch, J. (1992). *Thinking body, dancing mind.* New York: Bantam.

Khalighi. D. J. (1989). *Coming alive: The creative expression method.* Kentfield, CA: Tamalpa Institute.

Knaster, M. (1996). *Discovering the body's wisdom.* New York: Bantam.

Lefco, H. (1974). *Dance therapy: Narrative case histories of therapy sessions with six patients.* Chicago: Nelson Hall.

Minton, S. C. (1997). *Choreography: A basic approach to using improvisation.* Champaign, IL: Human Kinetics.

Olsen, A. (1998). *Body stories.* Barrytown, NY: Station Hill Openings.

Rosenberg, J. L. (1985). *Body, self, and soul.* Atlanta, GA: Humanics Limited.

Roth, G. (1997). *Sweat your prayers: Movement as a spiritual practice.* New York: Putnam.

Schoop, T. (1974). *Won't you join the dance?* Sedona, CA: National Press Books.

Siler, B. (2000). *The Pilates body.* New York: Random House.

Steinman, L. (1986). *The knowing body.* Boston: Shambala.

Todd, M. E. (1937). *The thinking body.* New York: Dance Horizons.

Wethered, A. (1973). *Movement and drama in therapy: The therapeutic use of movement, drama and music.* Boston: Plays.

Wosien, M. (1974). *Sacred dance.* New York: Thames & Hudson.

162   *Expressive Arts Therapy: Creative Process in Art and Life*

Therapeutic Drama/Myth/Storytelling

Allen, P. G. (Ed.). (1989). *Spider woman's granddaughters*. New York: Fawcett Columbine.

Blatner, H. (1973) *Acting-in: Practical applications of psychodramatic methods*. New York: Springer.

Boal, A. (1995). *The rainbow of desire: The Boal method of theatre and therapy*. New York: Routledge.

Campbell, J. (1968). *The hero with a thousand faces*. Princeton, NJ: Princeton University Press.

Campbell, J. (1988). *The power of myth*. New York: Doubleday.

Combs, G., & Freedman, J. (1990). *Symbol, story, and ceremony*. New York: Norton.

Emunah, R. (1994). *Acting for real: Drama therapy, process, technique and performance*. New York: Brunner/Mazel.

Estes, C. P. (1992). *Women who run with the wolves*. New York: Ballentine.

Larsen, S. (1988). *The shaman's doorway*. Barrytown, NY: Station Hill Press.

Polster, E. (1987). *Every person's life is worth a novel*. New York: Norton.

Gersie, A. (1997). *Reflections on therapeutic storymaking*. London: Kingsley.

Gersie, A., & King, N. (1990). *Storymaking in education and therapy*. Stockholm: Stockholm Institute of Education Press.

Houston, J. (1996). *Your mythic life*. San Francisco: HarperSanFrancisco.

Jennings, S. (1998). *Introduction to drama therapy: Theatre and healing*. London: Kingsley.

Jones, P. (1996). *Drama as therapy: Theatre as living*. New York: Routledge.

Krippner, S. (1988). *Personal mythology*. Los Angeles: Tarcher.

Moreno, J. L. (1947). *The theatre of spontaneity*. New York: Beacon House.

Pearson, C. (1991). *Awakening the heroes within*. San Francisco: Harper.

Remen, N. R. (1996). *Kitchen table wisdom: Stories that heal*. New York: Riverhead.

Røine, E. (1997). *Psychodrama: Group psychotherapy as experimental theatre*. London: Jessica Kingsley.

Rothenberg, J. (Ed.). (1985). *Technicians of the sacred: A range of poetries from Africa, America, Asia, Europe, & Oceana* (2nd ed.). Berkeley, CA: University of California Press.

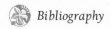

Shattner, G. (Ed.). (1980–81). *Drama in therapy*. New York: Drama Book Specialists. (Vol. 1—Children, Vol. 2—Adults)

Simpkinson, C., & Simpkinson, A. (Eds.). (1993). *Sacred stories*. San Francisco: HarperSanFrancisco.

Sparrow, G. S. (Ed.). (1980) *Awakening the dreamer*. Virginia Beach, VA: ARE.

Wethered, A. (1973). *Movement and drama in therapy: The therapeutic use of movement, drama and music*. Boston: Plays.

Walker, A. (1996). *The same river twice: Honoring the difficult*. New York: Scribner.

Williams, A. (1989). *The passionate technique: Strategic psychodrama with individuals, families, and groups*. London: Routledge.

Therapy and Music

Beaulieu, J. (1987). *Music and sound in the healing arts*. Boston: Station Hill Press.

Bonny, H. (1978a). *Facilitating GIM sessions* (GIM Monograph No. 1). Salina, KS: Bonny Foundation.

Bonny, H. (1978b). *The role of taped music programs in the GIM process* (GIM Monograph No. 1). Salina, KS: Bonny Foundation.

Bonny, H., & Savary, L. M. (1990). *Music and your mind: Listening with a new consciousness* (2nd ed.). New York: Harper & Row.

Borczon, R. (1997). *Music therapy: Group vignettes*. Gilsum, NH: Barcelona.

Bush, C. A. (1995). *Healing imagery and music*. Portland, OR: Rudra.

Campbell, D. (1989). *The roar of silence: Healing powers of breath, tone, and music*. Wheaton, IL: Theosophical Publishing House.

Campbell, D. (1991). *Music, physician for times to come*. Wheaton, IL: Quest.

Campbell, D. (1992). *Music and miracles*. Wheaton, IL: Quest.

Diallo, Y., & Hall, M. (1989). *The healing drum*. Rochester, VT: Destiny.

Gardner-Gordon, T. (1993). *The healing voice: Traditional and contemporary toning, chanting, and singing*. Freedom, CA: Crossing.

Hale, S. E. (1995). *Song and silence: Voicing the soul.* Albuquerque, NM: La Alameda.

Halpern, S. (1985). *Sound health.* New York: Harper & Row.

Hart, M. (1990). *Drumming at the edge of magic.* New York: HarperCollins.

Kenny, C. (1989). *Field of play.* Atascadero, CA: Ridgeview.

Kenny, C. B. (1982). *The mythic artery: The magic of music therapy.* Atascadero, CA: Ridgeview.

Kenny, C. B. (1995). *Listening, playing, creating: Essays on the power of sound.* Albany, NY: SUNY Press.

Keyes, L. E. (1973). *Toning: The creative power of voice.* Marina del Rey, CA: DeVorss.

Locke, D. (1992). *Kregisu: A war drum of Ewe.* Tempe, AZ: White Cliffs Media.

Lingerman, H. A. (1988). *Life streams: Journeys into meditation and music.* Wheaton, IL: Theosophical Publishing House.

Mathieu, W. A. (1982). *The listening book: Discovering your own music.* Boulder, CO: Shambhala.

Merritt, S. (1990). *Mind, music and imagery: Unlocking your creative potential.* New York: Penguin.

Ortiz, J. M. (1997). *The Tao of music.* York Beach, MI: Weiser.

Skaggs, R. (1997). *Finishing strong: Treating chemical addictions with music and imagery.* St. Louis, MO: MMB Music.

Steindl-Rast. D. (1995). *The music of silence.* San Francisco: HarperSanFrancisco.

Summer, L. (1998). *Guided imagery and music in the institutional setting.* St. Louis, MO: MMB Music.

Tame, D. (1984). *The secret power of music.* New York: Destiny.

Therapy and the Visual Arts

Adamson, E. (1984). *Art as healing.* London: Nicholas-Hays.

Arrien, A. (1992). *Signs of life: The five universal shapes and how to use them.* Sonoma, CA: Arcus.

Bayles, D., & Orland, T. (1993). *Art and fear.* Santa Barbara, CA: Capra.

Bonami, R. (Ed.). (1996). *Echoes: Contemporary art in an age of endless conclusions.* New York: The Monacelli.

Brooks, M. (1986). *Drawing with children.* Los Angeles: Tarcher.

Carbonetti, J. (1999). *The yoga of drawing.* New York: Watson-Guptill.

Case, C., & Dalley, T. (1990). *Working with children in art therapy.* New York: Routledge.

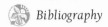

Case, C., & Dalley, T. (1992). *Handbook of art therapy*. New York: Routledge.

Craighead, M. (1986). *The mother's songs: Images of god the mother*. New York: Paulist Press.

Craighead, M. (1991). *The litany of the great river*. New York: Paulist Press.

Curtler, H. (1983). *What is art?* New York: Haven.

Dokter, D. (1995). *Arts therapies and clients with eating disorders*. London: Kingsley.

Dokter, D. (1998). *Arts therapists, refugees and migrants: Reaching across borders*. London: Kingsley.

Dockstader, F. J. (1961). *Indian art in America: The arts and crafts of the North American Indian*. Greenwich, CT: New York Graphic Society.

Edwards, B. (1979). *Drawing on the right side of the brain*. Los Angeles: Tarcher.

Edwards, B. (1986). *Drawing on the artist within*. New York: Simon & Schuster.

Fontana, D. (1994). *The secret language of symbols*. San Francisco: Chronicle.

Franck, F. (1973). *The Zen of seeing*. New York: Random House.

Franck, F. (1993). *Zen seeing, Zen drawing*. New York: Bantam.

Fürrer, P. J. (1982). *Art therapy activities and lesson plans for individuals and groups*. Springfield, IL: Thomas.

Gablik, S. (1991). *The reenchantment of art*. New York: Thames & Hudson.

Gablik, S. (1995). *Conversations before the end of time: Dialogues on art, life, and spiritual renewal*. New York: Thames & Hudson.

Gold, A. (1998). *Painting from the source: Awakening the artist's soul in everyone*. San Francisco: HarperSanFrancisco.

Goldberg, N. (1997). *Living color: A writer paints her world*. New York: Bantam.

Groenemann. (1994). *Through the inner eye*. Dubuque, IA: Islewest.

Henri, R. (1923). *The art spirit*. New York: Lippincott.

Hiscox, A. R., & Calish, A. C. (Eds.). (1998). *Tapestry of cultural issues in art therapy*. London: Kingsley.

Hogan, S. (Ed.). (1997). *Feminist approaches to art therapy*. New York: Routledge.

Howard, M. (Ed.). (1998). *Art as spiritual activity: Rudolf Steiner's contribution to the visual arts.* Hudson, NY: Arthroposophic Press.

Jennings, S., & Minde, A. (1993). *Art therapy and drama therapy: Masks of the soul.* London: Kingsley.

Kaufman, B., & Wohl, A. (1992). *Casualties of childhood: A developmental perspective on sexual abuse using projective drawings.* New York: Brunner/Mazel.

Kellogg, J. (1978). *Mandala: Path of beauty.*

Kellogg, R. (1969). *Analyzing children's art.* Mountainview, CA: Mayfield.

Keyes, M. F. (1983). *Inward journey: Art as therapy.* La Salle, IL: Open Court.

Killick, K., & Schaverien, J. (1997). *Art, psychotherapy and psychosis.* New York: Routledge.

Koff-Chapin, D. (1996). *Drawing out your soul: The touch drawing handbook.* Langley, WA: Center for Touch Drawing.

Landgarten, H. B., & Lubers, D. (Eds.). (1991). *Adult art psychotherapy: Issues and applications.* New York: Brunner/Mazel.

Liebmann, M. (1990). *Art therapy in practice.* London: Kingsley.

Linesch, C. (Ed.). (1993). *Art therapy with families in crisis: Overcoming resistance through nonverbal expression.* New York: Brunner/Mazel.

Lippard, L. R. (1990). *Mixed blessings: New art in a multicultural America.* New York: Pantheon

Little, M. (1997). *Miss Alice M and her dragon: Recovery of a hidden talent.* New York: ESF Pub.

London, P. (1989). *No more second hand art.* Boston: Shambhala.

Malchiodi, C. (1998). *Understanding children's drawings.* New York: Guilford.

Malchiodi, C. (1997). *Breaking the silence: Art therapy with children from violent homes* (2nd ed.). New York: Brunner/Mazel.

Markman, P. T., & Markman, R. H. (1989). *Masks of the spirit: Image and metaphor in Mesoamerica.* Berkeley: University of California Press.

McMurray, M. (1988). *Illuminations: The healing image.* Berkeley, CA: Wingbow Press.

McNiff, S. (1989). *Depth psychology of art.* Springfield, IL: Thomas.

Meglin, N. (1999). *Drawing from within.* New York: Time Warner.

Moon, B. S. (1992). *Essentials of art therapy training and practice*. Springfield, IL: Thomas.

Moon, B. S. (1997). *Existential art therapy* (2nd ed.). Springfield, IL: Thomas.

Rees, M. (1998). *Drawing on difference: Art therapy with people who have learning difficulties*. New York: Routledge.

Ridker, C., & Savage, P. (1996). *Railing against the rush of years: A personal journey through aging via art therapy*. New York: Mekler & Deahl.

Robbins, A. (1987). *The artist as therapist*. New York: Human Sciences Press.

Rubin, J. (1984). *The art of art therapy*. New York: Brunner/Mazel.

Schaverien, J. (1991). *The revealing image: Analytical art psychotherapy in theory and practice*. San Fransisco: Tavistock.

Schuman, J. M. (1981). *Art from many hands*. Worcester, MA: Davis.

Segz, L. (1976). *Masks of black Africa*. New York: Dover.

Simon, R. M. (1992). *The symbolism of style: Art as therapy*. New York: Routledge.

Skaife, S., & Huet, V. (Eds.). (1998). *Art psychotherapy in groups*. New York: Routledge.

Spring, D. (1992). *Shattered images: The phenomenological language of sexual trauma*. Savannah, GA: Magnolia Street.

Steiner, R. (1998). *Art as spiritual activity*. Hudson, NY: Anthroposophic Press.

Wadeson, H., & Durkin, J. (1989). *Advances in art therapy*. New York: Wiley.

Writing and Therapy

Adams, K. (1998). *The way of the journal*. Lutherville, MD: Sidran Press.

Baldwin, C. (1991). *Life's companion: Journal writing as a spiritual quest*. New York: Bantam.

Boice, B. *(1994)*. *How writers journey to comfort and fluency*. Westport, CN: Praeger.

Brown, R. M. (1988). *Starting from scratch*. New York: Bantam.

Cameron, J. (1998). *The right to write*. New York: Tarcher.

Capacchione, L. (1979). *The creation journal*. Athens, OH: Swallow Press Books.

Daniel, R. (1997). *The woman who spilled words all over herself: Writing and living the Zona Rosa Way.* Boston: Faber & Faber.

De Salvo, L. (1999). *Writing as a way of healing.* San Francisco: Harper.

Friedman, B. (1993). *Writing past dark.* New York: HarperPerennial.

Fox, J. (1995). *Finding what you didn't lose.* New York: Tarcher.

Fox, J. (1997). *Poetic medicine: The healing art of poem-making.* New York: Tarcher Putnam.

Goldberg, N. (1986). *Writing down the bones.* Boston: Shambala.

Goldberg, N. (1990). *Wild mind: Living the writer's life.* New York: Bantam.

Harrower, M. (1972). *The therapy of poetry.* Springfield, IL: Thomas.

Hinchman, H. (1997). *A trail through leaves: The journal as a path to place.* New York: Norton.

Hughes, E. F. (1991). *Writing from the inner self.* New York: HarperCollins.

Jerome, J. (1980). *The poet's handbook.* Cincinnati, OH: Writer's Digest Books.

Lamott, A. (1994). *Bird by bird: Some instructions on writing and life.* New York: Pantheon Books.

Lee, J. (1994). *Writing from the body.* New York: St. Martin's Press.

Lerner, A. (Ed.). (1977). *Poetry in the therapeutic experience.* New York: Pergamon Press.

Makin, S. R. (1998). *Poetic wisdom: Revealing and healing.* Springfield, IL: Thomas.

Mazza, N. (1999). *Poetry and therapy: Interface of the arts and psychotherapy.* New York: CRC Press.

Mezger, D. (1992). *Writing for your life.* San Francisco: HarperSanFrancisco.

Morrison, M. R. (1987). *Poetry as therapy.* New York: Human Sciences Press.

Oliver, M. (1994). *A poetry handbook.* San Diego, CA: Harcourt Brace.

Oliver, M. (1998). *Rules for the dance: A handbook for writing and reading metrical verse.* Boston: Houghton Mifflin.

Pearlman, M., & Henderson, K. U. (Eds.). (1990). *A voice of one's own: Conversations with America's writing women.* Boston: Houghton Mifflin.

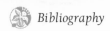

Progoff, I. (1971). *The star/cross*. New York: Dialogue House.

Progoff, I. (1972). *The white robed monk*. New York: Dialogue House.

Progoff, I. (1975). *At a journal workshop*. New York: Dialogue House.

Progoff, I. (1977). *The well and the cathedral*. New York: Dialogue House.

Progoff, I. (1980). *The practice of process meditation: The intensive journal way to spiritual experience*. New York: Dialogue House.

Rainer, T. (1978). *The new diary*. Los Angeles: Tarcher.

Sanders, S. R. (1995). *Writing from the center*. Bloomington, IN: Indiana University Press.

Strand, C. (1997). *Seeds from a birch tree: Writing haiku and the spiritual journey*. New York: Hyperion.

Walker, A. (1997). *Anything we love can be saved*. New York: Random House.

Dreams, Art, and Therapy

Bosnak, R. (1988). *A little course in dreams*. Boston: Shambhala.

Bosnak, R. (1996). *Tracks in the wilderness of dreaming*. New York: Dell.

Bulkeley, K. (1995). *Spiritual dreaming: A cross-cultural and historical journey*. New York: Paulist Press.

Campbell, J. (Ed.). (1971). *The portable Jung*. New York: Viking.

Campbell, J. (1988). *The power of myth*. New York: Doubleday.

Clift, J. D., & Clift, W. B. (1992). *Symbols of transformation in dreams*. New York: Crossroad.

Delaney, G. (1981). *Living your dreams*. San Francisco: Harper & Row.

Delaney, G. (1991). *Breakthrough dreaming*. New York: Bantam.

Dement, W. C. (1992). *The sleepwatchers*. Stanford, CA: Stanford Alumni Association Press.

Dombeck, M. B. (1991). *Dreams and professional personhood*. Albany, NY: SUNY Press.

Faraday, A. (1972). *Dream power*. New York: Coward, McCann, & Geoghegan.

Faraday, A. (1974). *The dream game*. New York: Harper & Row.

Freud, S. (1966). *The interpretation of dreams*. New York: Avon. (Originally published 1900.)

Garfield, P. (1974). *Creative dreaming*. New York: Simon & Schuster.

Garfield, P. (1979). *Pathway to ecstasy: The way of the dream mandala*. New York: Prentice Hall.

Garfield, P. (1988). *Women's bodies, women's dreams*. New York: Ballantine.

Gendlin, E. (1981). *Focusing*. New York: Bantam.

Gendlin, E. (1986). *Let your body interpret your dreams*. Wilmette, IL: Chiron.

Hall, C. (1953). *The meaning of dreams*. New York: Dell.

Hall, C., & Van de Castle, R. (1966). *The content analysis of dreams*. New York: Appleton-Century-Crofts.

Hill, C. E. (1996). *Working with dreams in psychotherapy*. New York: Guilford.

Hunt, H. T. (1989). *The multiplicity of dreams*. New Haven, CN: Yale University Press.

Jung, C. G. (1961). *Memories, dreams, reflections*. New York: Random House.

Koulack, D. (1991). *To catch a dream*. Albany, NY: SUNY Press.

Krippner, S. (Ed.). *Dreamtime and dreamwork*. New York: Tarcher.

La Berge, S. (1988). *Lucid dreaming*. Los Angeles: Tarcher.

Lauch, M. S., & Koff-Chapin, D. (1989). *At the pool of wonder*. Santa Fe, NM: Bear.

Linn, D. (1988). *The hidden power of dreams*. New York: Ballantine.

Mahrer, A. R. (1989). *Dreamwork in psychotherapy and self-change*. New York: Norton.

Mattoon, M. A. (1978). *Applied dream analysis: A Jungian approach*. Washington, DC: Winston & Sons.

Meier, P., & Wise, R. (1995). *Windows of the soul*. Nashville, TN: Nelson.

Mellick, J. (1996). *The natural artistry of dreams*. Berkeley, CA: Conari Press.

Moss, R. (1996). *Conscious dreaming*. New York: Crown.

Raffa, J. B. (1994). *Dream theatres of the soul*. San Diego: Luramedia.

Signell, K. A. (1990). *Wisdom of the heart: Working with women's dreams*. New York: Bantam.

Taylor, J. (1983). *Dreamwork: Techniques for discovering the creative power in dreams*. New York: Paulist Press.

Taylor, J. (1992). *Where people fly and water runs uphill*. New York: Warner Books.

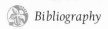

Tedlock, B. (Ed.). (1987). *Dreaming: Anthropological and psychological interpretations.* Cambridge, England: Cambridge University Press.

Tonay, V. (1995). *The creative dreamer.* Berkeley, CA: Celestial Arts.

Ullman, M., & Zimmerman, N. (1979). *Working with dreams.* Los Angeles: Tarcher.

Van de Castle, R. (1994). *Our dreaming mind.* New York: Ballentine.

Von Franz, M. L. (1987). *On dreams and death.* Boston: Shambhala.

Von Franz, M. L. (1989). *Dreams.* Boston: Shambhala.

Wiseman, A. A. (1989). *Dreams as metaphor: The power of the image.* Cambridge, MA: Ansayre Press.

Poetry for Ritual Use

Anderson, L. (1991). *Sisters of the earth.* New York: Vintage Books.

Bly, R. (1980). *News of the universe.* San Francisco: Sierra Club Books.

Rothenberg, J. (Ed.). (1985). *Technicians of the sacred.* Berkeley, CA: University of California Press.

Sewell, M. (Ed.). (1991). *Cries of the spirit.* Boston: Beacon Press.

Journals

American Journal of Dance Therapy
The Arts in Psychotherapy
Contact Quarterly: A Vehicle for Moving Ideas
Dreaming: Journal of the Association for the Study of Dreams
The Dream Network Bulletin
Journal of Art Therapy
Journal of Music Therapy
Journal of Poetry Therapy
Journal of the Association for Music and Imagery
Music Therapy
Music Therapy Perspectives
Poesis: A Journal of the Arts and Communication